M

28 DAY BOOK

HOW TO
PREVENT AUTISM

Copyright © 2017 by Dara Berger

Skyhorse Publishing books may be purchased in bulk at special discounts for sales promotion, corporate gifts, fund-raising, or educational purposes. Special editions can also be created to specifications. For details, contact the Special Sales Department, Skyhorse Publishing, 307 West 36th Street, 11th Floor, New York, NY 10018 or info@skyhorsepublishing.com.

Skyhorse® and Skyhorse Publishing® are registered trademarks of Skyhorse Publishing, Inc.®, a Delaware corporation.

Visit our website at www.skyhorsepublishing.com.

10 9 8 7 6 5 4 3 2 1

Library of Congress Cataloging-in-Publication Data has been applied for.

Cover photo credit Dara Berger

Print ISBN: 978-1-5107-1466-3
Ebook ISBN: 978-1-5107-1468-7

Printed in the United States of America

HOW TO PREVENT AUTISM

EXPERT ADVICE FROM MEDICAL PROFESSIONALS

BY DARA BERGER

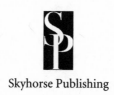

Skyhorse Publishing

This book is dedicated to the most special mother a girl could have:

Paula R. Silverman.

Thank you for planting the seeds in me many years ago with all those trips to the health food store. You were way ahead of your time.

I only wish we had the knowledge back then that we have today, so I could've helped you with your debilitating depression and food allergies.

I see your beautiful features in my children every day, and for that I'm so grateful. Some of your most precious qualities still live on inside me.

To my beautiful son Dylan,
your courage and unrelenting love are
a beautiful gift. I only hope that I have become
one half the amazing person you are today.

I would not have chosen our path, but this
powerful journey that we have been taken on
has inspired me to share your story in hopes
of helping others. Thank you for being my loving son.

I also dedicate this book to our other son
who we lost during my pregnancy with Dylan.

"I truly believe that if I were born today that I would have autism."

Disclaimer

This book contains the opinions and ideas of its author. It is written as a source of information only and not as a medical manual. It is sold with the understanding that the author and publisher are not engaged in rendering medical, health, or any other kind of professional advice or services to the individual reader. The reader should consult his or her medical, health, or other competent professional before adopting any of the suggestions in this book or drawing inferences from it. Neither the author nor the publisher shall be liable or responsible for any injury, loss, or damage allegedly arising from any suggestions or information in this book. Furthermore, the author and the publisher make no warranty, express or implied, with respect to the title or the contents of this book.

TABLE OF CONTENTS

ACKNOWLEDGMENTS

There are so many people and events in my life that came together to make this book possible to write.

My loving husband who feels like he is always last on my list will be thanked here first. He is one of my biggest supporters. There is no other person on earth who knows me the way that he does. Mark, you seem to know what I am thinking and feeling at times even before I realize it myself. You always encouraged me to go face the world, even at times when it was difficult to get out of bed. This journey that we have been on has been intense, but there is nobody with whom I would rather face the adversity and experience the happiness with. I love you with all my heart and being, even when we are nipping at each other. You will always be the greatest love of my life. Thank you for your friendship, kindness, and generosity. You have showed me that love can conquer all.

This book could never have been written if not for the love of my whole family. The relationship that I have with my beautiful daughter Jessica is one of the most healing ones I have ever experienced. There was a deep hole in my heart when I lost my mom, and I am so happy I get to give and experience with you what I did not have with my own mother. Thank you for holding such a special place in my heart. I love you more than words will ever tell. You inspire me each and every day. You are one of the most passionate and enthusiastic people I know. Guess the apple doesn't fall far from the tree! I have loved it each time you've asked me questions about this book project and told me how excited you were for its release into the world. My next book will be written with you, as promised, and we will teach as many children as possible how to experience real health like we have discussed so many times. I love you a million times over.

My brother, Scott, has been a great pillar of support for me while writing this book. He has read every word and given me helpful and constructive comments. There have been times when I have second-guessed myself and this project, and he has been there to remind me how important it is that the information in this book gets into people's hands no matter what and to put any insecurities I have aside. Thank you for your ongoing editorial/psychological support throughout this process. You have been there to remind me of how meaningful this project is to me on a personal level, given that I used to not even be able to read a book for the longest time due to my undiagnosed gluten allergy. I cherish our weekly talks, touching base about our lives, sharing the newest health information and, of course, discussing how crazy the world that we live in has become.

The support from my siblings has been so important to me, and I am blessed to have that twice over. My brother Mark has always been there on the sidelines, like a cheerleader cheering me on through all my endeavors. His protective big brother instincts have gotten me through some of the hardest times of my life, including acting as a parent towards me after we lost our mother. I feel enormous gratitude for having him as my sibling. He is always there to listen and never gets tired of hearing how hard it is to have a child with autism. I feel his immense support always around me.

I have been lucky enough to have many wonderful friendships over the years but one in particular sticks out when it comes to the writing process of this book. I met Kim Mack Rosenberg while we both volunteered our time for the National Autism Association New York Metro Chapter. She has been a wonderful confidante, someone I have so much fun with and, above all, a great supportive friend. She is always there to help with fact-checking, legal questions, and to discuss any personal issues with. Thank you for all your time and energy. You are a most special friend.

I have met some of the most incredibly dedicated people within the autism community. Many of them feel like family. Some of them are parents working tirelessly to advocate for all our children on the state level and trying to protect our children's rights. Others speak out about the harmful effects of vaccines in hopes of saving other children. Unfortunately, there are so many of us now, but I am thankful for their friendship and company. They hold my deepest respect.

I have chosen some of the brightest and most knowledgeable practitioners to give you the best and most up-to-date information on how to protect your child from autism. Each one of them took the time out of their busy schedules just so your child could have the life they deserve and be one less with autism. For that I am eternally grateful, as this book would not have been possible without each one of their participation. Thank you all for your devotion and passion in protecting all of our children!

Three mothers share their heartfelt journey. Thank you so much to Corrine, Katie, and Maria. There would be no way for people to truly get a picture of what it is like to have a child who suffers with chronic illness had you not shared your personal experiences with us. It took a lot of courage and respect for your child and all of us to do this.

Thank you to my publisher, Tony Lyons, for taking a chance on me as a first-time author. Many of us in the autism community highly respect you for the fact that you are not afraid to print books on subjects that are not so "mainstream." You will always have my gratitude for allowing us to reach so many readers and for giving us a voice to tell our story. A special thanks to Andrew Geller and Hector Carosso for all their hard work editing to make sure that the book sounded as clear and concise as possible.

Dylan's painful journey served as my motivation to compile the information in this book, in the hopes that others will not suffer the same consequences. I have dedicated this book to him, since it would never have been possible without our journey. There is an open letter to him at the end. I could never tell him enough how deep my love for him goes. It is infinite. I am not a particularly religious person, but I know God had a plan for us and we are fulfilling that plan each day. This book is part of that plan. I felt that something led me to this project for the last ten years. Our work is still not done. We plan to produce a documentary film on the subject, and I would love to write a children's book about health. Dylan, you did not suffer in vain. Your life experiences will help so many children for years to come all over the world. You have done such great work with your beautiful life. I wish I could handle things with the same amount of courage and grace as you have shown all of us. I am the messenger for your message. This book is your legacy.

FOREWORD
by Kim Mack Rosenberg

When Dara Berger first told me that she was thinking about writing this book, my immediate thought was that I wished a book like this had existed before I was pregnant with my son, who is now seventeen. Dara and I have known each other for many years. We met when we both began serving on the board of the New York Metro Chapter of the National Autism Association, but over time we have become close friends. Being an autism parent is rarely easy, but some of my strongest friendships (like that with Dara) have been forged in those fires. I knew a lot (though not all) of her personal journey, and I know how hard she has worked with both her children to make them the healthiest each can be. This book was borne out of her struggles and triumphs, seeking answers to help heal her son and to have a healthy second child. Her gift to you is the lessons she learned along the way, and the expert advice that she has brought together here to make your learning curve so much shorter than mine and hers have been!

There were, and still are, so many books on pregnancy and early childhood with messages that are, frankly, scary for parents-to-be and new parents, highlighting for them all of the things that can go wrong in pregnancy and early childhood development. I remember reading some of those books when I was pregnant and when my son was young and being completely stressed out—just what a mom-to-be or new mom does not need! In stark contrast, this book empowers parents-to-be by providing actionable preventative steps they can take before, during, and after pregnancy that may reduce the risk of their child being later diagnosed with autism spectrum disorder or other chronic illnesses.

The reality is that we live in a world where all of us are exposed to so many toxins, and some of us are more susceptible than others to the effects of those toxins. It would be easy to throw up your hands and give up, feeling like there is too much to overcome. To help readers from feeling overwhelmed and defeated before they even begin, Dara—and the experts she consulted—show us how easy it is to make positive changes that will make entire families, not just our babies, healthier.

Dara has generously and openly shared her family's personal journey in this book and, like many other parents of children with ASD or other challenges, I see pieces of my own and my son's story in hers. Dara shares her son's health challenges and the changes she made before having her daughter. But this book is so much more than the story of her family, as compelling as that story may be.

Dara has made her personal story a springboard to the advice of credentialed experts with an alphabet soup of degrees: MD, RN, PA, MPH, PhD, RDN, CDN, and more. These experts treat children with ASD and/or research of the science behind ASD causation and other health challenges. Between them, they have many decades of experience and can offer advice and guidance that is rarely accessible to most people who are not their patients. By drawing together experts from a wide variety of fields with many different perspectives, the book offers unique breadth and insight into autism and children's health in one volume.

Be prepared, you are about to engage in a deep dive about genetic mutations, other susceptibilities and environmental factors—and the interplay between genetics and environment—that may put some children at greater risk for ASD. You will learn about the biochemistry of autism and what happens when metabolic and methylation pathways, for example, are not functioning properly. Having some understanding of these issues is critical to understanding why sometimes simple changes to diet or lifestyle can have a tremendous, positive impact on health. The experts here share their knowledge in an easy-to-follow format, making the science accessible to all of us, and they offer practical advice on how to use that science to your own and your children's advantage.

Dara also takes the experts' information and provides concrete tips on how to make your own kitchen healthier, and how to make wiser and safer choices in personal care and cleaning products to create a healthier home environment for everyone. You will learn what things to consider taking out of your diet and your home and what things to consider adding in. As you will learn, even small, inexpensive changes can have a big impact.

Finally, Dara shares the stories of other parents who have a child with autism and "almost autism." You will see that these women are true warriors in the fight for their children's health. By reading this book and incorporating the information from it into your own life, you too are taking a step toward being a warrior for your children's health.

Having a baby should be a joy-filled and hopeful experience. This book provides knowledge that can help make the experience even more positive.

Know that there are so many things you can do (many without spending a lot of money) to improve the lives of your children. Learn from the experts and those of us who have gone before you.

If knowledge is power, then you are about to become a lot stronger!

Kim Mack Rosenberg
President, National Autism Association,
NY Metro Chapter

PREFACE

From time to time, I see young mothers pushing strollers and saying, "They all walk and talk," in the placating tones that we all use to assure one another that our children will be just fine eventually. My only explanation for this phrase still being used is they haven't seen firsthand the given current epidemics of childhood chronic illness; this is no longer true. As I sit down to write this book, the number of children in the United States diagnosed with autism is one in sixty-eight. This number comes from the CDC (Centers for Disease Control and Prevention), however most of us in the autism community know that the figure is very outdated as it comes from data of children born in 2004. The World Health Organization estimates that including obesity, 52 percent of children are diagnosed with chronic illness and, omitting obesity, the number is still as high as 39 percent. A newer, more alarming statistic by the CDC is that one in six children are diagnosed with a neurodevelopmental issue.

What is happening to our children? We can no longer deny that there is something happening. I am forty-five years old, and when I was growing up, the incidence of food allergies, ADD, learning disabilities, and autoimmune disorders were infinitesimal compared to today. For some reason, people have become incredibly complacent about discovering the cause of this suffering. I have channeled all my energy over the last year to bring you the best information from some of the brightest practitioners in an effort to create positive change from our trauma and hard-won experiences.

First, I will tell my family's story detailing everything that occurred with my son that led him to an autism diagnosis. As I pour over his medical files, looking back on the issues and developmental events throughout his infancy, the diagnosis is not surprising. It's all there in black and white and if you know the signs, as I do now, it would have been apparent to a practitioner knowledgeable about chronic illness that he was headed towards a state of autism. Subsequently, I'll explain everything that I did differently through my second pregnancy with my daughter Jessica, beginning with cleaning out for three years. I definitely took it much further than one might need to, but I already had a child at home who had been suffering for years. I wanted to do absolutely everything in my power to prevent the same debilitating illness from striking our family twice. Please keep in mind that I am not a doctor or medical professional and most of what you will hear from me comes from my decade-long journey of personal research and experience.

The chapters following our personal experience contain valuable information from passionate and experienced practitioners who have spent their entire careers studying childhood chronic illnesses—especially autism. Each day they wake up and try relentlessly to help and heal those afflicted. I am honored and privileged to be given the opportunity to interview them for you. I love that despite their different areas of focus, they are all aligned on one important issue: the risks of autism can be greatly minimized, if not completely prevented by taking some simple steps and preventative measures. Some of them have treated my children and others have not. I have the deepest respect for the important work they do as well as their tireless devotion.

I purposely wrote this book so that you can read any chapter in any order, even if you choose not to read the book from cover to cover; each stands on its own. There is also a summary at the end of each chapter for your review. I am hoping that you find the information in this book very helpful for both yourself and your offspring. I can tell you from my own experience that it's extremely helpful when the whole family embarks on a healthy lifestyle together.

I include links throughout the chapters and towards the end of the book to different websites that contain helpful information or areas that you may want to investigate further. I encourage you to look at them, since they contain a wealth of information, including details that I may not have been able to cover as thoroughly. Finally, I hope you continue educating yourself about holistic health long after finishing this book!

PART I

CHAPTER 1

DYLAN'S STORY

I woke up every morning for the first two years and started crying before my feet even touched the floor. The first thought on my mind was, "I can't believe he still can't talk." The next thought was, "I can't believe he still has autism." It felt like a scene from "Groundhog Day," each day starting in exactly the same way, except I didn't get to learn French or how to ice sculpt. This wasn't a movie, this was my life and I was beyond devastated each morning. I used to drag myself from the bed to the bathroom and literally have to give myself a little pep talk. I would look into the mirror and initially think, "I just can't do this anymore." Then I would speak out loud, while pointing to myself in the mirror and say, "You can do this. You have to do this. If you don't do this, then who will." And I would stay in that bathroom until I was ready to say, "Okay, I can do this." There were days that it took a long time to muster those words and other days that I just faked it, going about my day like a robot. To say the pain was immense would be an understatement. There were actually times in those first two years that I stood on Broadway right outside my apartment and for a split second looked up at the oncoming traffic and thought, "I just cannot take this pain for one more second."

Lucky for me, those thoughts were very short-lived and I knew I just needed to get through that moment. Sure enough, I would feel better minutes later. The reason I include these very private and painful feelings that not even my husband was aware of at the time is to show you the extent to which the pain was just beyond measure. There is no way to quantify how upsetting it is to have a child become trapped in autism. For me, it was like he was dying a little bit every day while he was on his downward spiral. Then, once he finally bottomed out, it was hard to recognize that this was still my little boy other than the fact that he looked like my son. I felt completely helpless to stop him from slipping away a little bit more each day.

Another vivid memory from that time is of having dreamt every night that I was in the middle of the ocean drowning. Now it doesn't take a psychiatrist to figure this one out. I was drowning every day, all day long. It felt as if I was treading water out in the open sea with no land in sight. I was exhausted in every way possible: physically, mentally, and emotionally. It's amazing to me that I made it through with my marriage still intact. I think this experience has forced my husband and I to connect on a level we never imagined was possible. I remember just a few weeks ago, we took my son to look at a new school and I explained what I thought of it afterwards. My husband remarked that he already knew. He went on further to say that he feels like we can have a conversation without speaking just by looking into each other's eyes. And he is absolutely right. I attribute some of this to having a nonverbal son for seven years while we tried feverishly to restore his speech. We had no choice but to become very attuned to nonverbal language, since it was Dylan's only way to communicate for almost seven years.

My description of the debilitating pain of having a child diagnosed with autism is intended to instill a sense of immediacy to do all you can to prevent it. Autism is not like many other diseases or conditions in that your child either loses function or shows delay over three areas: cognitive, physical, and social. It can be very difficult to reverse autism once it gets going and, for some, the brain can be so severely impacted that full recovery may not be possible. This is the reason prevention is paramount. In my son's case, we have been working tirelessly to recover him for the past ten years and have made huge inroads. He has not yet recovered, but I thank God every day that we were able to restore his speech. It was through the help of some of the practitioners in this book that we were able to accomplish this high task. Dylan still has a long way to go and I will never give up on him, nor will his practitioners. Each practitioner has taught me the important lesson of leaving no stone unturned, and sometimes you even need to go back to the same stone and lift it up again.

In order to understand how to prevent autism, one must discuss what types of things might be causing it. There will be many discussions throughout this book on different causes of autism by professionals who hold different positions in the healthcare field, including doctors, scientists, nutritionists, physician assistants, and nurses. I chose a wide range of experts to give you a wide variety of perspectives on preventing this complicated and debilitating illness. What makes autism so difficult to understand is that there is no one factor that precisely causes it, and on the flip side, no one antidote that can reverse it. Scientists and practitioners study every single aspect of a child's life beginning in utero to see if they can pinpoint the things that may be contributing factors as a way to lower the risks in other children and to find interventions that may help that child recover. I have combed through every little thing Dylan has ever experienced to try to uncover what may have contributed to his autism in order to prevent it from happening to his sister. It can be painful to discover things that you did, which seemed harmless and innocuous at the time, only to realize that it was one piece in the puzzle that may have built up over time, damaging their little body. These discoveries are also important knowledge to have after the fact in order to help decide which treatments might be beneficial in undoing the damage.

HERE IS DYLAN'S STORY:

We tried to get pregnant for the longest time and it just wouldn't happen naturally. I had no idea at the time that I was truly not healthy enough to conceive a child. This is a concept I understand extremely well now, but the concept was foreign to me over ten years ago. Like most people, I didn't connect the dots that the way I lived my life had any bearing on my health, since I had been taught that what I ate and the products I used had absolutely no consequence.

My husband and I began trying to conceive a little over a year after we got married. At the time, everyone one around us seemed to be getting pregnant with ease, or so we thought. It was becoming particularly upsetting as anytime I went anywhere someone would ultimately ask me when I was planning to have a baby, as if I could just pick one up at the store. Additionally, people weren't openly discussing fertility issues as they do now. Nobody warned me how difficult the process can be for some people and what a strain it can put on your marriage when it doesn't happen so quickly. We endured so many months of "baby sex" (intercourse with the sole intent to get pregnant), which can place a huge damper on your romantic life, to say the least. There also wasn't anyone to explain that it could take years to recover from this kind of mechanical lovemaking. We decided to get some professional help with our fertility issues and experienced a few failed artificial insemination attempts before my gynecologist and fertility expert discovered that there was a polyp acting like a natural IUD. We had it quickly removed and then moved straight towards IVF. I was really tired of trying to have a baby—no, actually I was exasperated with the process. To say I felt immense pressure to get pregnant would be the biggest understatement of the year. I felt tentative about the idea of using hormones, but couldn't shoot myself up quick enough with those IVF drugs. I had to get my baby. The desperation was palpable.

Lucky for me, I was able to get pregnant on the very first try. I still remember how scared I felt during those two weeks after the embryos were transferred and all we could do is wait to see if any of them took. You can't help feeling helpless when things are completely out of your hands; much like how I feel while I wait each day to see if the next treatment I try works and cures my son's autism. I was immensely thankful when I was told it seemed like two embryos took. It felt like all my suffering was paying off, and things in my life were finally going right.

However, this excitement would be short-lived, given that my OB was very honest by disclosing during my first ultrasound appointment that it looked like only one seemed strong enough to make it. This was one of those juxtaposed moments, where you receive great and horrible news at the exact same time. I was ecstatic at the reality that I was finally pregnant, but secretly sad in knowing that there was a good chance one of my babies would not make it. I tried to stay positive, thinking that maybe the weaker one could hang on. Sadly, my positivity didn't change the reality that only one viable embryo showed up on the ultrasound two weeks later.

I felt very sad at the time but did not really speak to anyone about it, not even my husband. It wasn't until very recently that I started marking "yes" to miscarriage on medical forms. I had never really acknowledged it, since we never felt the embryo was really ours given that we were told so early on that it probably wouldn't make it. Our baby never grew enough to have a heartbeat or any of its specific organs. But I now realize that I lost a baby and Dylan lost his twin sibling. My life is much richer for finally finding a place in my heart for this event. My husband and I even talked about the possibility of naming him Paul after my mother Paula. It seems like such a funny thing to make such a big acknowledgment about something so many years later, but I cannot express to you how right it feels.

There were many other things about my pregnancy with Dylan that were also not so simple. When I look back at his brief two years of life before the bomb dropped out of the sky with the autism diagnosis, it's not easy to point to any one thing that caused his illness. Like many of the professionals you will hear from throughout this book, I believe there are many things that build up over time and then something ultimately pulls the trigger. The contributors that build up and the trigger are very different for each child. However, once you have traveled down this road, the things that contributed become very apparent in retrospect, and this information is very helpful in choosing the most useful treatments to try to recover your child. It is also equally as helpful in preventing autism in your next child. You have the knowledge to avoid these things the next time around. My understanding and recognition of many of these contributors and signs to look for is the sole reason I have a healthy and completely neurotypical six-year-old girl. Some kids are just lucky, but in my daughter's case, I worked my ass off to make it happen. Or, I should say, not happen. And the work started years before I ever thought of getting pregnant again. My plan is to one day tell my daughter how her brother took a bullet for her for all of us.

I am thrilled to have the opportunity to share my experience and the wealth of information that I have collected over the last ten years, so that you too can prevent autism. But it won't just stop there, you can apply this information to prevent many other chronic childhood illnesses. You will also be able to prevent disease in yourself, or begin healing an ongoing illness. I find it most helpful to work with a highly qualified practitioner, especially while embarking on this new, healthier lifestyle. A nutritionist can be helpful in making dietary adjustments over time, whereas a functional medicine doctor or naturopathic doctor may conduct specific tests to uncover possible nutritional deficiencies and imbalances that need to be addressed.

I'm extremely proud of my battle wounds. However, I would never have chosen this journey, since this would mean that I chose for my son to suffer. I am not sure that he would say the same thing, since he is such a beautiful giving soul. He may have asked for autism if given the choice, so that his baby sister would not suffer the same fate. He is the most courageous person I have ever met. Dylan will always be my hero. Until recently, I did not think it was possible to love him anymore than the day he was born.

I will never forget the exact moment he was born. My husband was adamant about not finding out the gender, and kept saying this is one of the few times in life that it will be a wonderful surprise either way. How could I argue with that? Secretly I kind of wished for a girl; I wanted to have that girl companionship, which may be as a result of losing my mom at such an early age. I never got to have that wonderful mother/daughter bond as she was abruptly taken from me at thirteen years old.

I finally gave birth to my son after an extremely unnatural childbirth that I will go into further detail later. The doctor announced that I had a boy, inside I was momentarily bummed. Moments later they took my son over to the table to be examined, which included a lot of poking and prodding. They finally brought him to me after what seemed like an eternity, and gently placed him in my arms. I remember that I looked down at his little innocent body with those huge, gorgeous blue eyes staring back at me and it was love at first sight. I fell in love with him in an instant. It was pure magic! It was one of the happiest moments of my life, evident from the huge gleam in my eyes in the pictures that my husband took in the delivery room that day.

I wish that I could say that we lived happily ever after, although this could not be farther from the truth. Dylan's stay in the hospital was pretty uneventful, so they let us go home after only thirty-six hours. It would be years later before I recognized how incredibly healthy he was given that he was born five and a half weeks early. His Apgar was an eight and nine out of ten and he was breathing on his own without any difficulty, which was considered a sign that he was extremely healthy. Many babies born that early, including the child of a couple we shared a room with right before the delivery, need assistance to breathe and are put in the NICU for several weeks. Dylan was the picture of good health. The only thing out of the ordinary was immediately following the birth, they took him from us for around twelve hours to keep him under the lights, since he was born with a little jaundice. The hospital considers this completely normal given that it is so common. I, on the other hand, wish I understood that this may have been his very first sign.

As I mentioned earlier, one of the biggest signs was that I could not get pregnant. I was not healthy enough to procreate. In fact, I was suffering from a horrible autoimmune illness referred to as multiple chemical sensitivities, which is basically a state of being allergic to almost everything around you. And yes, I am being quite serious. I used to have to smell a book before I could purchase it, since I was allergic to the different kinds of inks that are used in printing. It even got to the point where I couldn't sit next to someone on a NYC bus who was reading the newspaper. It was that bad. My biggest fear at the time was that I would get trapped in an elevator with someone wearing too much perfume. At one point, I really thought that I was going to have to leave NYC and live out the rest of my life in a log cabin. Luckily for me this didn't happen, but my story is not uncommon in being a mother who suffers from a chronic illness prior to getting pregnant and has a child who goes on to be diagnosed with autism. Basically, I am saying that my own illness already stacked the deck against Dylan. This was a pretty big contributor, but it's still only one of many as I later discovered. The practitioners I interview will also mention that it's fairly common to hear that mothers of children diagnosed with autism were suffering from some sort of chronic illness or allergies prior to their birth such as Crohn's disease, asthma, depression, or fibromyalgia. An even more interesting fact is that the same contributors that lead to the child's autism diagnosis are some of the same things that resulted in the mom's condition.

Next on my list of contributing factors would be IVF. I will never forget the day I asked my wonderful and caring OBGYN what the risks were in doing IVF.

His answer was so simple and unlike most doctors. He told me that there could be overstimulation of my ovaries and that we have no idea what the long-term effect of these drugs are, or if they cause cancer. This was one of the first doctors for whom I ever developed the deepest respect and trust. That was eleven years ago, and I don't believe any safety studies have been performed on the subject to date. Most women, including myself, are so desperate to get pregnant that the safety concerns would never even cross our minds.

I wonder a lot about what exactly was in those multidose vials I used during my IVF treatment. Sometimes I even consider sending some remaining, unopened medication off to get tested, especially to see if there are heavy metals present. There needs to be some kind of preservative when you are sticking multiple needles in the same container. I want to say for the record that I am not against IVF or those medications, I am merely sharing all the contributing factors that may have played a part in Dylan developing autism, including my own chronic illness at the time of the pregnancy. Now that I have given my disclaimer, let's get back to Dylan's story.

Once I was able to get pregnant, there were plenty of other "not so great" influences on him. First, I was on antibiotics during the first trimester for a tooth infection at about ten weeks gestation. I will let the doctors explain in more intricate detail why this can result in a problem and the things that you should do if you find yourself in need of antibiotics. Next, I was exposed to fumes coming from my neighbor's renovations in the apartment one floor below ours. He was painting his whole apartment using very strong smelling oil-based paints and refused to open his windows even once he was aware of my pregnancy. Unfortunately, he was very callous about the whole matter. At my insistence, my husband and I eventually moved out of our apartment after a few days and stayed in a hotel nearby for the duration of the work. However, I will never know what breathing in that smell during the first trimester may have done. We got the building manager very involved and he was helpful in forcing this person to give the building all his plans in advance, as well as access to his apartment so the windows could be opened. It may have been a little too late. Again, this is just another "contributor" at a vulnerable time in Dylan's development. This also occurred at around ten to eleven weeks into the pregnancy, a very delicate time when the fetus is still developing all of its organs.

The rest of my pregnancy seemed to be pretty run of the mill until the third trimester when my OB went on a trip, referring me to one of her colleagues while away. I will never forget when the receptionist handed me the other doctor's business card, she told me to bring a lot of reading material due to the fact that this physician triple booked. I remember thinking, "That doesn't sound so great." I wondered, "Why am I going to see them?" Well, not great turned out to be one of the biggest medical mistakes. Not only did I wait for hours as I had been warned, but then she barely gave me any time during the appointment. She seemed much more interested in hearing what I did for a living than checking on the health of my baby. And I wouldn't discover the worst thing that she did that day until weeks later. She made a horrible error when she neglected to check my urine. This is one of the most important things an OB can do to a pregnant woman, especially in the third trimester. I started to really not feel well in the days after and finally ended up in the emergency room in preterm labor due to an undiagnosed urinary tract infection. I was admitted and given IV antibiotics. All the doctors and nurses prepared me for the fact that I might deliver Dylan at thirty and a half weeks. This was devastating news for someone as careful as me. "How could this even happen to me," I thought, "when I was just at the doctor's office?"

I felt fortunate for sustaining the pregnancy and not to giving birth to Dylan during that horrible week-long hospital stay. Instead, after much begging and pleading with my doctor, I went home and spent the next four weeks on bed rest before I finally gave birth to him at thirty-four-and-a-half weeks. During that period, there was tremendous stress between my husband and me, as he had to play the role of my caretaker and continue to fulfill all the day-to-day requirements at his job. To make matters worse, the second round of antibiotics to treat the UTI were even stronger than the first dose, since it was given intravenously. This became another BIG contributor, as it wiped out all my good bacteria so that when Dylan finally came down the birth canal, he did not inherit the diverse balance of good and bad bacteria of my gut flora that is essential to building a healthy immune system. We will refer to this collection of good and bad bacteria as the microbiome. In essence, I feel it was as if Dylan was born by cesarean section. This is another risk factor that we will explore throughout the book with various practitioners who will offer some helpful and important suggestions on how to deal with this situation should it arise for you.

Besides antibiotics, the hospital also gave me certain pharmaceutical medications such as Ambien, since I found it hard to go back to bed when a nurse woke me up each evening in the middle of the night to take my temperature and blood pressure. After a few nights, I decided that I no longer wanted to be taking the sleeping pills that had probably never been tested on pregnant women, and I asked my doctor to stop having them wake me up at 3 a.m. for unnecessary tests. She realized that it did appear ridiculous when I laid it out for her. The point here is that you need to be a detective, as well as your own advocate. If something does not make sense to you, then don't agree to it.

Despite these early negative influences, Dylan was able to meet many of his milestones generally on time. Some, such as smiling, were a little bit late. He was very alert with an extremely healthy appetite. Unfortunately, my milk never really came in, so we were forced to supplement with formula. I was never crazy about store-bought formula, considering I could barely pronounce any of the ingredients. I remember thinking, "What other choice do I have?" It didn't seem like there were any other options at the time. The next time around with my daughter, I not only learned of other options but also created my own.

Dylan did start to develop some physical symptoms when he was just seven months old, such as a yeast rash around his penis that was relentless and wouldn't go away. This was another sign that something wasn't quite right with his immune system, which I only recognize in hindsight. Pediatricians will tell you it's totally normal, since every kid has it at some point and Dylan's run of the mill doctor was no different. But you wouldn't consider Parkinson's normal because everyone had it. Next came the eczema, where I was offered another prescription cream to mask the symptom and not fix the underlying cause. Then there were the constantly red cheeks that my pediatrician kept saying was dry skin. She had me slathering Aquaphor on his face all day and night, even though it did nothing. What I find sad is that it's actually well known that red ears and cheeks are an obvious sign of food allergy. Most pediatricians still miss this every day—unless they are holistically minded. He was also spitting up large chunks of formula; yet another overt sign of food allergy that was completely overlooked. I will let the practitioners go into much greater detail about this topic and the importance of early recognition.

I wanted you to see that all the signs were there if someone knew the road map to autism. Vaccinations were the straw that broke the camel's overloaded back for Dylan, and I share our experience in greater detail in that chapter. Again, there are many other triggers that can catapult a child into the abyss of autism. There are also numerous smaller stressors and contributors that we will discuss, such as pesticides and chemicals in our cleaning and personal care products. All it takes is for these smaller contributors to add up and meet the trigger when the body is feeling vulnerable or has just had enough! They refer to this as the total load theory.

Chapter 2

THE DIAGNOSIS AND AFTERMATH

It was one of those beautiful, crisp, still, perfect New York City fall days, except this one would turn out to be one of the worst days of my life. It was the day that changed everything. You look back over the years and remember certain moments in your life that stick out, especially those that are pivotal in defining the rest of your life. This one was one of those moments.

My husband and I took Dylan to a neurologist on the Upper East Side that was recommended by our pediatrician. He examined Dylan for an extremely short period of time, maybe just a few minutes and then asked us to sit down right before he dropped the A-bomb on us. That would be the autism bomb. He only used the word once during that fateful visit and then referred to Dylan's diagnosis the rest of the time as PDD-NOS, otherwise known as pervasive development delays. Most doctors do not like to diagnose children under three years old with autism in case they "grow out it." I will never forget that he stood up to shake our hands and give us his business card and then said, "There is no cure, but some find a type of therapy called ABA helpful." I remember standing there frozen in time in shock, not being able to say anything or move any of my limbs. I thought, "How could this be?" How could my beautiful little boy have a horrible illness that this doctor is saying has no cure.

Somehow I found the strength to shake his hand, gather our things, pay the bill, and get myself back out to the car. I remember my husband asked me where I wanted to go shopping once we were all settled in the car. I replied that I didn't want to go anywhere and that I was not expecting the doctor to say autism. My husband replied, "Did he say that?" I bluntly answered, "What doctor's office were you just in?" He laughed and said, "Denial, I guess." At that moment, we both started laughing hysterically, you know the nervous in-shock kind of laugh. But I knew in an instant that we were going to be okay, that I would somehow survive this if I could laugh with him at one of the worst moments of my life.

When I look back now what is even more upsetting to me than that doctor giving me the "there is no hope speech" were the appointments with my pediatrician leading up to that day. My husband and I definitely had some concerns that Dylan's speech was not developing properly and he tended to get easily upset or overwhelmed around a lot of people. The turning point was after a week-long stay in Long Beach Island, New Jersey, with my brother and his family. During this trip, Dylan cried whenever my brother's three sons tried to play with him or were running around chasing each other. This was upsetting for me to watch but on the other hand, we were also pretty used to this behavior. My brother made it a point to call me up when we got back home and insist that I bring him to see a developmental pediatrician. This was pretty jarring for me to hear, but I knew that he was saying it in my best interest and he was not getting off the phone with me until I promised to make that appointment with a specialist. I was upset with his implication that something was wrong with my beautiful baby, but nonetheless complied, given that he had a lot more experience than me with already raising three children who were older than Dylan. Secretly inside I did not feel that everything was perfect with him, even if I did not fully admit it to myself or to my brother. Unfortunately, the only appointment with this specialist was six weeks out, so in the meantime I thought it would be prudent to bring him in to the pediatrician's office to get her take on everything. This would prove to be another huge mistake.

Dylan and I had an appointment with the pediatrician a few days later and arrived at her office on time as usual. She was running particularly late that morning and kept us waiting for about forty-five minutes, which is your typical nightmare when you have a two-year-old in tow. When she finally entered the room, it seemed like she was in a big old rush and never really made eye contact with either of us. She sat at her computer, typing away the whole time while I relayed that we had serious concerns about his language development. I was never asked any important questions that would have been a huge red flag such as, "Has he ever had language and lost it?" or, "Does he only repeat words or utterances after someone has just said them?" Instead she turned to me and said, "New Yorkers are crazy, he will talk. You just have to be patient and nobody likes to wait anymore." To this day when I think about her statement, I get angry at her incompetence and wonder how many other children she has hurt and done this to since that day. But in that moment, I had a false sense of relief since I felt she was the professional and I trusted her. It never dawned on me that not only did she express what I wanted to hear, but she did my son a gross injustice by not fully examining him or the issue during that appointment.

I pulled out my phone to call my brother the moment I exited the doctor's office to tell him the good news that there was nothing wrong with my son. Instead of sounding relieved, he was incredibly angry to hear that our concern was dismissed and that I had already just cancelled the appointment with the well-known developmental pediatrician. I promised my brother in that moment that I would still consider making another appointment with the specialist to make sure everything was really okay, even though I felt confused given that our pediatrician seemed confident that there was nothing to worry about. She was supposed to be the expert.

Flash forward two weeks later when I brought Dylan back again to see the same pediatrician for a two-year-old well visit, in which she actually took the time to spend more than two minutes with us, and she told me he needed to be evaluated immediately. I was beyond angry with her in that moment. How could she make such a flip-flop after I cancelled that appointment just two weeks prior. I know she felt like some kind of idiot when I received a phone call late that night telling me she personally called the neurologist's office asking if he could fit us in in the next day or so. Unfortunately, this experience of mine is not uncommon and still exists to this day. I did extensive volunteer work for the National Autism Association New York Metro Chapter for six years, starting with its inception and had an incredible amount of contact with hundreds of other parents who had children on the autism spectrum. It's shocking how often I heard this same story repeated back to me over and over. It's an incredible shame that most pediatricians don't know or recognize the early signs before it results in a diagnosis of autism or developmental delays. And to make matters worse, many of them dismiss what turns out later to be valid concerns. When a child is treated early, the outcome is so much better since you are in essence preventing autism before it actually happens. This is the sole reason that I have chosen to write this book, so you can learn to recognize these early signs before things snowball and your child eventually gets diagnosed with some horrible chronic illness.

I won't pretend that life was easy in the days and weeks after that doctor's visit. The truth is the following two years were some of the darkest days of my life. And it's not like adversity had never touched me before. I had lived through my mother's suicide at thirteen years old and somehow thought that that would be the hardest thing I would ever have to go through. Boy was I wrong—since nothing will ever hold a candle to how difficult having your child diagnosed with autism can be. My son abruptly lost the ability to speak overnight and he had to learn how to climb stairs again, which felt like it took forever. It wouldn't be until years later that I would learn that he actually had suffered an ischemic stroke, which is not uncommon after vaccines. My son also had no ability or idea how to play with toys appropriately and no longer looked me in the eye. As I mentioned earlier, I cried every morning when I woke up for the first two years. It was beyond anything anyone could ever imagine. He was alive but trapped in a body that no longer worked. He continued regressing for a long time after his autism diagnosis. I was under immense acute and chronic stress, since his illness affected every part of my life and seemed to be enveloping us. Every moment became centered around managing his illness. They say that the stress mothers who have a child of autism experience is similar to that of a combat soldier. I tried very hard to lead a normal life by continuing to go to the gym, see friends when I could, but it was so difficult to ignore how many things in my life had been altered.

My son could no longer do all the things that a typical child could and neither could I. I lost friends, my independence, an enormous stress was put on my marriage, and most of all there was very little joy left in life with the constant worry that we would never be able to fix him. My days were spent either in front of the computer or a book researching ways to get him better, making doctor appointments or going to a seminar to learn about some new intervention for children with autism. Life was sheer hell, but I never stopped believing that one day I would get him better. Dylan and I were trapped in the house all day with constant therapy starting at 9 a.m and ending at about 6 p.m. It felt like I was in the witness protection program, since we both became virtual prisoners to his illness.

I feel grateful that we were referred to a functional medicine doctor and nutritionist very early on by the developmental pediatrician who noticed he was self-limiting his food to eating only dairy and gluten. In the visit with his first functional medicine doctor, Dylan was diagnosed with the works: gluten and dairy food allergy, fatty acid deficiency, heavy metal exposure, gut dysbiosis, and hyperactive immune system. I started him on an extensive biomedical protocol that day, which included probiotics, fish oil, vitamins, and a special diet.

I will always remember when Dylan's first biomedical doctor, Nancy O'Hara, mentioned to me in those early visits about cleaning out before having another baby. She explained that it was something that she did before she had her son. I was nowhere near ready to even think about having another baby since the very thought would create immediate panic, but I never forgot that conversation. I must have filed it away in my brain under important things to remember.

A few months later, I made an appointment with one of the other doctors in her practice who treats adults and I was diagnosed with all the same things as Dylan. As they say, the apple doesn't fall far from the tree. My protocol got me better within nine months and I am happy to report with a lot of effort, I no longer suffer from any autoimmune illness. Dylan's autism truly saved my life. And this would only be the first life he would save, as he would go on to help so many others. I have shared his story with so many friends, cousins, even his therapists at school to keep them from suffering the immeasurable pain of having a child diagnosed with autism. It was only after the countless families Dylan has helped that I had an epiphany that we need to do this on a much larger scale, so we could reach many more people. I consider this book to be Dylan's legacy, taking all his pain and suffering, using it to hopefully help hundreds and thousands more children. I may have written this book on paper, but I consider myself just the medium for Dylan's message on how vital prevention is, especially in today's toxic world.

Over the next few years, Dylan and I went on many different diets including a gfcf (gluten- and casein-free) diet yeast-free diet, and SCD (specific carbohydrate diet). The specific carbohydrate diet helped Dylan a lot by healing his digestive tract and making him calmer. Although Dylan made strides on this diet, it proved miraculous for me as my allergies were down 70 percent in just the first six weeks on the diet, which is why I stayed on it for another three years as part of my clean-out process in case I would go on to have another baby one day. This diet is also referred to as a grain-free diet and is considered extremely healing for the gut. Everything you eat is a whole food that you cook yourself, since no processed foods are allowed. Suprisingly, even my husband gave up his twice a week pizza habit and went on this diet with us, experiencing many improvements such as lowering his cholesterol ten points and losing roughly thirty pounds. We did everything as a family together and this was no exception as life was just so much easier when we all shared the same eating habits.

Dylan and I also did many other natural/therapeutic interventions together such as B12 shots, vitamin-C IV's, chelation, homeopathy, Homotoxicology, herbal supplements, hyperbaric soft chamber, helminthic therapy, and the list goes on. My progress was always much quicker than Dylan. I wished to God it could have been the other way around. If you told me that I could give my right arm for Dylan to be better, I would have said, "What are you waiting for? Take it now!"

Dylan lost his language literally overnight from a vaccine reaction at eighteen months old and did not speak again for the next seven years. Doctors and therapists told us they were not sure that he would ever speak again. I refused to accept this notion and put all my faith in the healing process. I truly believed that something happened to him, putting him in that state and felt there must be a way to bring him back. I am happy to report that we finally were successful in getting Dylan talking four years ago when he was eight and a half years old. People look at me shocked when I mention this to them, especially speech therapists or other professionals that regularly work with children on the spectrum. Unfortunately, many doctors and our media report that these children cannot recover, which is so far from the truth. Some children get better just by doing a gluten-free diet, and for others it's rather slow like watching an iceberg move as in Dylan's case. And then some kids are so damaged that they barely show any progress over the years. I know how absolutely heartbreaking and devastating it can be to try treatment after treatment with no positive outcome. Many parents find themselves crying on their child's birthday, since it is a reminder that another year of their childhood is gone, and I am no exception. Although I am less sad each year given all the progress he has succeeded in making, I know in my heart that Dylan is a happy kid, but I can't help but feel that he has missed his whole childhood trying to get better. The childhood he was supposed to have.

I honestly wasn't even sure that I would be able to go through with having another baby. The mere thought of doing this again with another baby could almost produce a full-blown anxiety attack. You hear plenty of stories about families who have two, three, or four children on the spectrum. I have even met my share of them, but I still don't have any idea how they do it. They are my true heroes.

During this time when I was trying to get Dylan and myself better, all my friends around me were popping out their second or third child including some of my friends with special needs children. They would pressure me with questions every time I saw them about when I was going to have another child. Everyone knew what I was attempting to do as far as cleaning out to ensure a better outcome with the next pregnancy, but nonetheless I would be made fun of. They made jokes about my diet, since I was refraining from eating gluten and processed food. There was no secret that I was scared to death to have another baby. The truth is I wanted one more than anything in the world and each day I would ask myself if I was clean enough to have one yet.

This long journey of cleaning out lasted about three years until I finally felt confident enough that my body was in a much better state. It would have been less stressful if someone would have just handed me a certificate that I had completed the necessary requirements for having a healthy baby. Unfortunately, I was in unchartered territory and there was nobody else I knew who was doing or talking about this concept. As I mentioned earlier, I won't take credit for coming up with the idea. It was again Dylan's first functional medicine doctor, Nancy O'Hara, who spoke to me about the concept of cleaning out. I basically took the idea and ran with it for three years with the help from some very dedicated practitioners, including Geri Brewster who is also featured in this book.

This cleanout process also entailed doing food allergy testing to see what foods I might be allergic or sensitive to. This is how I realized that I had a condition, which is now referred to as non-celiac gluten sensitivity. Taking gluten out of my diet was literally a miracle for me. I always felt cloudy with an impaired memory and had no reading comprehension or word recall. Once I gave up gluten, I could read up to two books in a day and my memory became almost photographic. It always amazes me how I got through school with decent grades with this gluten disability that I had my whole life. Next up was a stool test to see how I was digesting my food. When you have a child on the autism spectrum, you begin to realize that your microbiome (also referred to as the balance of good and bad bacteria in your gut) is your most prized possession in helping you to stay healthy and keep chronic illness at bay. I also did extensive blood work each year that gave me clues into how my body was compensating for things that were going on such as nutritional deficiencies, malabsorption, and gut dysbiosis, not to mention my own lifetime accumulation of toxins that we will refer to as the mother's body burden.

I was working so hard towards getting to the point where I could feel comfortable with the idea of getting pregnant again, except there was nobody to tell me that I was finished. My mind was plagued by insecure thoughts that maybe I was still toxic or hadn't done enough. I just wanted desperately for someone to tell me that I had done the necessary work and was clean enough to carry and have a healthy baby. As you know, there is no crystal ball to give you this information. I guess a part of this is hard work, dedication, and a leap of faith that you have done all you can.

Chapter 3

JESSICA'S STORY

Dylan was five years old when I turned thirty-nine, and I thought to myself, "It's now or never." I made a promise to myself that I wouldn't beat myself up if it did happen again, since I was doing everything in my power to try to prevent autism. Shockingly, we got pregnant on the very first try. This was a fabulous sign that I was finally healthy enough to procreate. I immediately made a list of everything that I was going to do differently this time around, including a natural childbirth, maybe even with a doula or midwife. My husband was so excited and dizzy hearing about all my plans every second of each day, especially when I would come out to the breakfast table first thing in the morning and cite all kinds of studies from PubMed before he even had a sip of coffee.

I immediately consulted with my functional medicine doctor and nutritionist about all my ideas regarding which supplements I needed to take, food I should eat during the pregnancy, including my childbirth plans. I split my day down the middle by tending to my son's illness, trying to find new therapies and interventions to help him get better, and at the same time researching and planning ways to have a healthy child. It would be accurate to say that I lived and breathed pursuing both of these passions for my son and unborn daughter.

As I've said, I was extremely careful during my second pregnancy. My husband would probably describe me as being obsessed. I would leave nothing to chance this time. My plan was to have a natural childbirth with very little medical intervention. I was careful with my diet, continuing all my supplements during the pregnancy such as probiotics, fish oil, vitamin D3, methylfolate, multivitamin, vitamin C, etcetera. Endless hours were spent researching the safest crib, mattress, and clothing made from the greenest materials. I read book after book on natural childbirth, hired a doula, and took a hypnobirthing course.

Another major thing I did differently was to call my OB and ask her if she was affiliated with the same doctor that made the mistake of not diagnosing my urinary tract infection. I found out that indeed they still worked together in the same group practice, so I explained that I would not be using her for this next pregnancy. My thinking was that I could not bear to get stuck in a labor and delivery room with someone who already caused me and my son so much pain and suffering.

I was very lucky to have chosen an open-minded OB this time around. For instance, she was very tolerant of me for not wanting to drink the sugar drink that they give all pregnant women to check for gestational diabetes, and instead gave me a full endocrine blood work up. I told her one time that we were not going to speak about vaccines, since I had a previous reaction to a tetanus shot and my son suffered a devastating stroke after a routine vaccine when he was eighteen months. She immediately dropped the subject, honoring my request and pretty much left me alone until the beginning of the third trimester. In the beginning of the third trimester, I measured 6 cm dilated in one of my exams. She wanted me to go on bed rest for the next three to four months, which I declined after extensively going over every detail that everything else was perfectly healthy with the pregnancy including the absence of any contractions including Braxton Hicks. Every time we spoke, she tried to convince me that I might have the baby in an elevator with no time to get to the hospital. This didn't make sense, since I wasn't having any contractions. I carried on with my life for another three to four months with no babies being born in the elevator. At forty-one weeks, she told me I would have to be induced if I did not give birth to my little girl over the weekend. I smiled, appeased her, and said of course, knowing full well that I was not getting induced unless the baby was in danger. I knew that I had a great amount of fluid and my daughter was strong. And besides, forty-two weeks used to be the norm to have babies until it got changed to forty weeks. It just didn't make sense to me not to be patient a little bit longer and wait for Mother Nature to do her thing. My little girl was fine and I was going to sit tight until she was ready to make her grand entrance. I believe doctors are too used to controlling things and there was no viable argument for forcing the delivery to happen on Monday. It was such an arbitrary thing to pick that day, like picking a number out of a hat.

I checked in with my doula a few times a day at this point. There were a few false alarms when I went to the hospital a couple times not sure if I was in labor. It was difficult to know when I was in actual labor since I never had a normal labor the first time around with Dylan and my OB was placing immense pressure on me to have the baby soon or I would continue to be talked into getting induced. One time I sat with my husband in the car for two hours outside the hospital and then we turned around and went home. I didn't want to be stuck in the hospital labor room if I was not in active labor. Once you get admitted to a hospital and you are not in labor that's when they try to really speed things along by bringing out all the bells and whistles, such as an epidural, Pitocin, forceps, episiotomy, and, God forbid, a C-section. There have been some interesting theories out there linking Pitocin and epidural as possible contributors to autism. Nothing is definitive, but my thought was, "Why take a chance?!"

During one of these false alarms, I actually got examined in the triage area and they told me that I was still only 6 cm dilated. They brought me to a room and asked me to change into a gown, then moments later came back and announced that I should be admitted. I asked them if I was in active labor and the doctor again said no, so I told her and the nurse that I did not want to stay. She tried to coerce me by saying that it was dangerous to go home, which really wasn't true being that I was still the same 6 cm dilated that I had been for over four months. She told me that she was going to leave the room so I could think about it, in which time I took off the gown and got dressed while the doula and my husband watched. The doctor came back in the room and, as my husband would describe it, she looked like she saw a ghost. I told her that I was going home until I progressed further, but promised I would come back at the slightest change. My doula was supportive and my husband got a little freaked out that I signed something that said I was leaving against medical advice. I was like, whatever—I am not having another traumatic childbirth and being forced into interventions that I have no interest in subjecting my beautiful healthy baby to.

I went home and nothing out of the ordinary happened that night or the next night. Then on Saturday, I went back up to the hospital not sure if the contractions were strong enough to be in labor. Once again, I was examined and still was only 6 cm dilated. I knew that this going back and forth to the hospital was a result of my OB's pressure that I would need to get induced after the weekend if I did not give birth. I would be lying if I wasn't still slightly annoyed describing what stress she had put me under. Immediately after the exam, I was in tremendous pain and I told this to the attending doctor. She kind of acted like she didn't know what I was talking about. I persisted further, describing that I had never been in that kind of pain following a pelvic exam. It was then that she admitted to giving me a very aggressive exam, which I thought was awful. It never hurt so much to urinate in my life and she could have hurt my baby just to rush me along into labor. Unfortunately, this type of action is not uncommon.

I went home that night and awoke a few hours later to being in labor and knowing it for sure this time. There was no mistaking it. My husband took me back to the hospital where we met the doula again. She was so patient with me and happy that I was standing up for myself. This time I let them admit me, giving the administrator all my paperwork that I brought with me including a notarized document stating that I did not want any vaccines given in the hospital and a note from my pediatrician saying that he wanted our newborn baby to be given oral vitamin K at birth as opposed to the standard vitamin K shot, which has many contraindications including death listed on the package insert. I think most people do not even know that when they bring your baby over to the table to weigh them that they get this shot automatically. I think it is unnecessary, considering most European countries give the vitamin K orally and have no increased problems with blood clotting. The vitamin K injection is not without risks. You can read the package insert online to decide for yourself.

After finishing up the admission paperwork, they led me to a delivery room, while walking down the hall I breathed a sigh of relief that I was finally going to have my natural childbirth. When I entered the room, I could not believe my eyes when the same doctor that delivered my son was right there in front of me. I was completely traumatized in that moment, feeling a wave of post-traumatic stress come over me. All I could think is, here is the doctor that tortured me the first time around during Dylan's birth. I wanted to dash out the hospital door, only this time I couldn't leave since I was actually in labor with intense contractions that were progressing rather quickly. So I made the decision in that instant I would stand my ground and not allow her to do anything I didn't want, no matter what (barring an emergency).

She fought me on wanting to stand up next to the fetal monitor machine so I could move around during the contractions. However, I did not give in and stood next to the machine while I hunched over a pillow on the bed during the contractions. At one point, she came in and told me that the fetal heartbeat was falling and I would have to start pushing even though I was only 8 cm dilated. I immediately remembered something from one of my books that said to change positions if the heartbeat goes down at any point. So I looked at her and said, "I am just going to stand up for a moment." What do you know, the fetal heartbeat immediately went back to normal. She just kind of looked at me dumbfounded. I remember screaming silently in my head, "How could she not know this?" I read so many great tips just like this one in a book called *Gentle Birth Choices* by Barbara Harper, RN. She probably single-handedly saved me from having my vagina ripped apart by this doctor who wanted me to push before my body was ready.

I stayed in labor for about one more hour before the happiest moment occurred and this doctor's shift was over. The sign of relief I felt could never accurately be described in words. Nothing has ever made me happier than to see that doctor vacate my delivery room. I then started to cross my fingers hoping that her replacement wasn't going to try to make me do anything that would put me or the baby in danger. And she didn't. Actually, it was a breath of fresh air that she was the exact opposite. This new doctor basically had one of her nurses with me the whole time and stayed out of the room until right before I was about to give birth. At one point, I was actually nervous that there was no doctor in the room and I was bent over in agony. The nurse was amazing and brought me a squatting bar that gets attached to the bed, so that gravity can help facilitate the birth the way nature intended. They were all there supporting my natural childbirth experience. I remember at one point right before my daughter was born, I looked the doctor in the eye and said, "I can't do this." She looked at me like a deer in the headlights, but luckily a moment later her natural instincts kicked in and she began cheering me on like a football coach. This is another common experience that the book *Gentle Birth Choices* describes happening. My beautiful baby girl was born just moments later. We named her Jessica Sara Berger.

I did everything differently this time, proving that you can have a hospital birth and stay away from harmful interventions if you work hard at it. I held my daughter close right after she was born and began trying to breastfeed immediately, which was so different than Dylan's birth. I did what felt natural and she instinctively knew what to do. We bonded in such a precious way that I actually felt high for like three days after her birth. I always tell people that it was my Mount Everest. It is such a shame to me that so many women will never experience what I felt that day and in the days after, the most beautiful experience of my life. We are taught to fear the experience rather than allow it to empower us. I have already begun talking to my six-year-old daughter about how beautiful her natural childbirth felt to me in hopes she does not grow up to fear it for herself.

Unfortunately, immediately after the birth, my elation was followed by aggravation. The nurses wanted to take my daughter to the nursery to bathe her. I did not want to be separated from her, my biggest concern was that they would vaccinate her or do some other intervention that I did not want. They told me they had to take her. I said that I wanted to be with her at all times. This went back and forth. Finally, I blurted out in an exasperated tone, "Then I will leave the hospital with her now and go home." Everyone in the room was completely silent. And they all looked at me in utter shock including my husband and the doula. But I was dead serious and they all knew it. There was no mistaking that I knew my rights as I rattled off the New York State Patient Rights booklet that the hospital gives you like ten times. I had the right to leave the hospital and the right to say no to any treatment or intervention. They knew I was not backing down and finally relented, taking me in a wheelchair with my daughter to the nursery so I could watch them bathe her. Next, she accompanied me to my room where we stayed for the next two days. Every time the pediatrician on staff needed to check my baby, they came into the room and politely asked me to accompany her to the nursery.

I accomplished everything I set out to do and could not be happier with the results. My daughter Jessica is a beautiful, sassy, artistic, hyper verbal, humorous, and most importantly a very healthy little girl. This is not to say that we did not experience some bumps in the road of her development, and for this reason I dedicate a whole chapter in the book to this concept of looking for and dealing with early signs that something is amiss.

Here are some of the bumps in the road that we experienced with my daughter: Jessica developed a dairy allergy very early on, which once again was stressful given that there are not a lot of options out there. I had no choice but to take milk out, even though at the time she was receiving most of her calories from formula. I consulted with an extremely intelligent nutritionist who helped me build a homemade baby formula using hemp and coconut milk. I had already tried the Weston Price Foundation liver–based option that Jessica refused to take. The nutritionist was very careful to make sure that Jessica was getting the required and recommended amount of nutrition and calories that her growing body needed. Once again, I was in unchartered territory as I had never heard of anyone doing a hemp and coconut milk formula, including my experienced nutritionist who specializes in working with families that have children on the spectrum. She was more than willing to diligently work hard to help me create this special formula for my daughter, given the other options contained so much junk including genetically modified foods, chemicals, and preservatives, and tons of corn syrup. We ended up perfecting a formula that Jessica stayed on for the next five months.

Then at around eighteen months, we started to notice that she was still not walking and talking, while beginning to appear more frail. Naturally, I was frightened beyond belief that she too might be headed toward a state of autism. There was not an ounce of denial. I had already taken her to get a speech evaluation at nine months old, and subsequently started to receive speech therapy four times a week. I don't think I slept a wink for weeks while I tried to uncover what was wrong with her. We had expensive blood testing done including an ion from an independent lab, which basically looks at everything, and your neurotransmitter levels. We got back a surprising answer that Jessica had lead poisoning. You must be thinking, what kind of a mom am I that could allow this to happen. Well it's not so simple how it occurred. Our pediatrician was so shocked that he repeated the test before telling me about the lead and he confirmed that the first test was indeed correct. This would explain a lot about her present state of delays at the time. However, Jessica had no sign of lead six months earlier at her twelve-month visit, which included a standard blood test for lead.

This was one of the scariest moments of my life. I was in shock but had no choice except to figure out what to do next. There was no time to waste being upset. I made an appointment with four of the smartest doctors and nutritionists that I knew, some of which have been interviewed for this book. Each of them had a different suggestion, which confused me even more. And to make matters worse, I felt tremendous pressure to do something right away. My instinct guided me to take a deep breath, listen to my gut, and take some time to figure out the best possible option. I felt it was better to do the right thing at the right time than to act too hastily and regret your decision later on. Sometimes you only have one time to get it right and this felt like one of those times. Scott Smith was the practitioner that suggested we use vitamin C, which most people don't know chelates heavy metals, plastics, and pesticides from the body. I figured why not start with the most gentle and natural protocol, and if it doesn't work out, I can always move on to the stronger suggested regimens. And it was like a miracle. She started to walk within two weeks of taking the vitamin C and began speaking four weeks later. Each time I followed Scott's protocol and raised the dosage, the progress could be seen immediately. It was truly amazing and I believe even Scott was surprised at how quickly it worked. Jessica's therapists who were treating her at the time had never seen a child make that kind of progress that quickly.

A year later she developed eczema, which I took very seriously, since that type of T2 dominance of the immune system can lead to a more serious illness like asthma if left untreated. We gave her herbal supplements such as uva ursi and aloe juice to treat the underlying inflammation, leaky gut, and gut dysbiosis that were the causes of most of her issues. We will talk more about this concept in detail later in the book.

Many of Jessica's symptoms are similar to the ones Dylan experienced, such as the eczema, food allergies, and heavy metal poisoning. We never did find the cause of the lead poisoning even after testing our water, dust, and toys extensively. I have resigned myself that it may be part of my body burden that was passed down to her in utero. They say the best way to chelate a woman is for her to have a baby. It's horrible but true that we pass on our accumulated toxins down to our child while they are in the womb. Studies show that they find more than two hundred chemicals in baby cord blood when it's tested. You cannot protect your child from every little thing in this world, however you can thoughtfully consider the best and safest way to handle what you cannot prevent.

I feel grateful every day for her good health and take nothing for granted, nor do I ever let my guard down. There are many other illnesses that are milder and less debilitating that a child can develop besides autism. So I continue my work to prevent all of them in order for her to be happy and enjoy her childhood, rather than experience sickness during it.

These days I find myself desperately trying to strike an even balance between allowing her to live a little and trying to be a good mom in keeping her healthy. This is no easy task. If it were up to her, she would eat carbs and sugar all day long. I always remember that it is my hard work and pure diligence that has paid off allowing her to have a normal childhood. I also have a constant reminder with my son's autism how things can be if I let loose too much. I continue to cook three meals a day for her and keep track of the amount of undesirable food that she eats such as pretzels, popcorn, or potato chips. This may seem daunting to you, the constant looking over your shoulder for autism, but the flip side is so much more exhausting and devastating. I promise you that there is nothing worse than looking on helplessly as a neurological disease ravages your child's body and holds them hostage for years, as it has done to my son. Autism has robbed him and hijacked his childhood.

As a country, we are ill-prepared for what many experts refer to as a tsunami of adult children with autism who are about to age out of the system that supports and takes care of them. The burden will now be on local state and city municipalities. And a bigger threat is that autism has not been presented fairly and openly, so most Americans don't have any understanding about what is coming down the pipeline. They read in newspapers how these children are all a little quirky, but somehow they go on to college and lead very productive lives. Our media is quite guilty of only portraying the positive image of a child with autism being allowed to play basketball and making that three-point shot with five seconds left to go in the game leading their team to victory. The general public just has no concept that this is a rare minority and that the majority of children on the spectrum have huge behavioral, cognitive, and physical challenges that greatly impact their day-to-day functioning. Parents many times find themselves forced to quit their job so they can stay home to properly care for their child that may be experiencing one hundred to two hundred seizures a day. Did you ever notice how the sizes in diapers have changed over just the past decade? Many children with autism never go on to be potty-trained or do any other basic self-care things such as feeding themselves or bathing, even when they become adults. So, if you think that embarking on a healthier lifestyle would be more difficult than changing your adult child's diaper in a public restroom, then maybe this isn't the right book for you.

PART 2

CHAPTER 4

WHAT IS AUTISM?
with Sidney Baker, MD

Let's begin with the acknowledgment that there is a problem that we are trying to prevent. The rates of autism today are astronomical compared to even just a couple decades ago. Back in the 1990s, it was estimated that around one in two thousand children were diagnosed with autism, as opposed to our present-day figures, which the CDC now estimates is one in sixty-eight children. However, most people don't know that the data for that figure was taken from children born in 2004. Essentially, that number is already twelve years old. Logic dictates that the current number of diagnoses will be exponentially higher.

For many years, the sentiment was echoed over and over again that this increasing incidence was just better diagnosis, which may be true in a small percentage of the cases. However, this does not explain the near meteoric rise. I begin each interview with the same question of whether the rates of autism have been increasing, and each practitioner offers their own unique perspective.

Recently, we have started to hear the word neurodiversity used a lot more often in conjunction with autism, which is currently being used to justify that autism has always been around. The question remains that if autism was always there, then why are books being written on the subject, since it would be so obvious to everyone and not newsworthy enough for publication? Secondly, those of us who have been involved in the autism community for many years would like to know where all these adults with autism have been hiding all these years because, as a society, we are just starting to see the influx of young adults now. By influx of young adults, I mean that as a society, the population of children who were born in the '90s—when there was a sharp increase in autism incidence—are just aging out of the education system and becoming adults. They were the first generation of kids in the beginning wave of the explosion in autism.

Another indicator of the increasing rates of autism is the implementation of new training programs for first responders (police, fire, medical, etc.). Again, if autism has always been around, then why the need for these training programs since we would have all grown up surrounded by individuals who meet the medical requirements for a diagnosis of autism, and therefore would theoretically be well-equipped to manage people with autism or the symptoms of autism without the need for new training programs. I merely mention this as a point of contention, as there have been so few efforts made to recognize the urgency and severity of this issue by the media, our government, or among the medical community. Many of us in the autism community feel that there is a huge amount of denial in recognizing that we have an epidemic going on.

Genetic causation theories have also been floated, but professionals studying genetics have debunked this theory as a sole cause, given that historically there has never been a genetic epidemic in existence. This is not to suggest that there isn't a relationship between genetic mutations and an increased risk of autism; but rather that genetic predispositions are not the "sole cause," as some might suggest. There have also been many lesser-known theories, such as the mother's or father's age at the time of conception and many others, none of which have ever been proven to be valid.

Well, the good news is that professionals in the autism community have been studying this causation issue as it relates to autism for years. This movement started when a group of doctors got together from the Autism Research Institute to compare notes and created one of the first autism conferences for parents to learn about cutting-edge treatments for autism, and to give training to doctors on how to help heal those children affected by autism with biomedical treatments, such as B12 shots, glutathione, and gluten-free dairy-free diet. Dr. Sid Baker, whom I interview in this chapter, was one of the founding members of what was formerly called the Defeat Autism Now! Conference, and has been a long-standing advocate of increasing public awareness surrounding autism, it's diagnosis, treatment, prevention, etc.

So, what is autism? A simplistic way to conceptualize autism is it is a collection of symptoms showing a delay across three specific areas: social, cognitive, and physical. While this conceptualization may be helpful in understanding autism from a general perspective, unfortunately it isn't particularly informative in assisting individuals with autism manage their diagnosis, helping parents develop treatment protocols for their children, or guiding medical professionals to pinpoint and treat specific symptoms unique to each patient's "autism." When my son went for his evaluations over a decade ago, my husband and I were told that he presented with a certain percentage delay across all three of these areas. Some of the symptoms of delay might include poor eye contact, low muscle tone, delayed speech, lack of reciprocity (inability to be socially and emotionally connected to another individual), and the inability to follow simple commands. If you ask most parents of children with autism what the word "autism" means, they will tell you it's an upsetting word that doesn't represent much of anything. Meaning, it's kind of like saying someone has cancer—but not specifying what kind, what body part is affected, or what stage it's in.

Additionally, many children with autism often have comorbid conditions, which means that they have two diseases appearing simultaneously. For example, a child might present with a seizure disorder and apraxia (inability to speak) concurrently, whereas another child might have mitochondrial dysfunction and hypotonia (low muscle tone). Moreover, children with autism often present with more than just two conditions at any given time, including my son. Unfortunately, no two children are alike, which makes developing a singular treatment or prevention protocol extremely difficult. Nobody knows exactly what causes autism, but we do understand what things contribute to it. We also know how to help the body stay in balance (i.e. homeostasis) and heal itself, meaning there are a multitude of necessary preventative measures to protect against autism and other childhood chronic illnesses.

Another important concept is that most chronic illnesses are caused by the same underlying issues. The factors that are believed to trigger autism are generally the same for most chronic health issues. Throughout this chapter, Dr. Baker and I will begin to touch on many of the things that contribute to many autoimmune illnesses, but especially in the case of autism.

Dr. Sid Baker began his career as a faculty member at Yale Medical School where he received his medical training and specialty in pediatrics and a mini-residency in obstetrics, after which he served as a Peace Corps volunteer in Chad, Africa. Additionally, he is the former director of the Gesell Institute of Human Development in New Haven, Connecticut. Dr. Baker has maintained a general practice for many years, where he has treated both adults and children with complex chronic health issues—including many children with autism. He has also written several books including *Autism: Effective Biomedical Treatments, Detoxification and Healing: The Key to Optimal Health*, and *The Circadian Prescription*.

Dr. Baker was highly instrumental in helping me restore my son's speech— as he recommended a certain type of therapy that was very successful with

Dylan when all other treatments fell short. I send people with some of the most difficult chronic illnesses, such as Parkinson's or Alzheimer's, to him. He is a passionate and creative soul who will leave no stone unturned, who will never stop looking for answers, and who will never give up on you or your child.

DB: Is there an increase in autism?

SB: No doubt about it. It's amazing to me that people are struggling to accept that conclusion, even today. For example, we see new books published each year that advocate all kinds of explanations about how autism was always there, it's not new and it's not increasing. Frankly, that's nonsense. It's interesting how people can come to this conclusion considering that the data is now very solid discounting all these other factors—like genetics and a better diagnosis.

There's a vast, alarming increase which is matched by increase in all kinds of problems in young and old people, the vulnerable edges of the age distribution where there is something going on because it's not genetic. By nature of the process of evolution, genetic mutations are an inherently slow process—and therefore the conclusion that a genetic epidemic has occurred in the case of autism is a fallacy at best. It must be that something is going on in the environment that's affecting individuals on epidemic proportions. There's not only an increase, but there's a credible reason for why that increase is coming about—because something in the environment is changing humans' immune system and nervous system.

DB: What is autism for people who don't know anything about it?

SB: I think it's important to steer clear of the traditional explanations of autism, in terms of the behavioral problems: problems maintaining eye contact, speech, and the like; these are symptoms of autism, they don't define autism. When we talk about autism, I think what's really 'wrong' is the loss of tolerance, as it relates to one's senses. There are twelve senses; not just five as most people presume. So in essence, when we're talking about people with autism, we're talking about the inability to tolerate certain kinds of stimuli that a majority of the population can handle.

Managing sensitivity is something that is a joint effort of the immune system and the central nervous system. Whereas the central nervous system takes care of the world around us on a macro-level, the immune system takes care of the invisible world of molecules. While these two systems examine and process different aspects of the world around us, they are alike with respect to our capacity to tolerate the world.

DB: You have a long history of treating many children with autism. How did you first come to get involved with autism?

SB: In the early 1970s, I was an attending physician in an institutional setting in New Haven. This was a part-time job doing the physical exams and the routine medical work there as well as being on call. I was asked to do a physical exam on an autistic boy. And despite seeing hundreds of patients between my daily practice and my work at the institution, this was my first acquaintance with a child that had autism. There I stood at the end of the examining table to begin my physical exam from the top down with the normal routine of looking into his eye with my ophthalmoscope. As I drew near, he slugged me right in the middle of the bridge of my nose. My failure to have removed my glasses before using the ophthalmoscope revealed my nervousness and he took them off all right [he laughs]. My glasses went flying in two pieces, and I thought to myself, "Oh my god, what he did was a spectacular feat of precision." Only later did I realize that his speechless gesture was an eloquent way of saying, "You are looking into me but you are not seeing *me*." It got me thinking!

DB: You have a very different way of treating people as individuals. Could you explain how you first started treating patients with bio-individuality?

SB: I took what is now called a "gap year" between my junior and senior year at Yale. I spent three months with an American doctor, Edgar Miller, in Kathmandu, Nepal, who would look at me after each patient that we saw together in his little clinic and say, "Sid, have we done everything we can for this patient?" When I went to medical school after that, the question was, "Have we done everything we can for this disease?" The focus on the patient was already branded on my heart, so I was stuck with the notion that the patient is the target of treatment. Then, when I became a practicing pediatrician and family doctor and I listened to my patients, their stories further validated Dr. Miller's question.

DB: How would you describe your current practice?

SB: My family practice turned into what I might call "resort medicine." People say, "What resort do you work at?" I say, "The last resort." I see people with complex chronic illness. I've learned about that from many of my intelligent friends and teachers along the way, and have consistently followed this path that started with what Dr. Miller said to me in Nepal, which is the patient is the target of treatment. Everybody is different. The same treatment doesn't necessarily work for the same diseases.

DB: Tell me the story of the little girl that you treated many years ago. She was the first child that experienced a recovery from autism because of your treatment.

SB: A little girl came to me with eczema all over her, and the eczema emerged within a week of taking some antibiotics. A neighbor who knew me said, "You should go see Sid because he knows about the antibiotics and the eczema." So she came to see me and I said, "Yes, I think you have a yeast problem: a candida overgrowth because of the antibiotics killing your normal germs, and if we give you a little Nystatin™, it should probably help with the eczema." This was just a quick visit for the eczema. She went on the Nystatin™ and the eczema cleared up completely, *so did her autism.* [Pauses] She was autistic. I thought, "Oh my god, now this is getting heavy." So that was the beginning of my engagement with autism. I had recently become the director of the Gesell Institute, where my interest in information technology led me to focus on autism. That focus was on the details of each child's symptom profile, as opposed to just the symptoms that led to the autism label.

DB: You told me about an experience you had in medical school with your first introduction to autism that really shocked you. Can you expound on this?

SB: I was taught many things in medical school, most of which I've forgotten. But one lesson that resonated with me was during my time at the Yale Child Study Center as a second-year medical student. They showed us a movie with a dignified physician sitting behind a big mahogany desk. [He points.] Over there were mom and dad, parents of a child who was out of the room. The message from the doctor was,

"Well, George and Jane, I'm terribly sorry to tell you that Johnny has a problem that is not going to get better. The thing that I think you really should understand most critically is not to look for answers." I was stunned because I was sitting in medical school hearing a lot of new stuff. I was stunned and it took me a while to absorb those words. Even when you have terminal cancer, you can go to Sloan Kettering Hospital and they say, "Well we have a protocol. We have something, we can try." I couldn't wrap my head around why doctors at the Yale Child Study Center (and presumably elsewhere around the country) could hold the position of "don't look for answers." I was shocked by that.

The ideas presented to me about autism other than it being an inborn thing that we couldn't do anything about was to blame it on the mother. This was a tragic mistake in medical thinking. This resulted in the child being separated from the mother and they would administer psychotherapy to the mother and put the child in an institution. Later in the 1970s and '80s, I met families who had suffered from this misaligned thinking back in the 1970s and '80s. This destroyed families. It shows you how wrong the experts can be.

DB: What causes autism? Can you talk a little bit about what we think contributes to autism?

SB: We think that it has to do with the fact that our environment has become contaminated with substances, which are not good for us. When I say "not good for us," I'm not only referring to lead and mercury—old-fashioned toxins in industry and commerce—but novel chemicals too, such as dioxins, polychlorinated phenols, herbicides like Roundup, and so on. The human system has been acquainted with toxins of various kinds throughout our evolution. We, like all living things, have systems for ridding ourselves of our own waste molecules and toxins that come from our food and environment. However, in the last hundred years, the burden of novel man-made toxins on humans' health and well-being has exploded.

DB: Why are these toxins a problem now?

SB: The total load, as we call it, overburdens our body's task of proverbially "taking out the trash." It is a key function in our chemistry that is central to many activities that overlap with the chemistry of growth and making new molecules. The same chemistry that's involved in fixing up your DNA when it's broken, or changing your DNA when it needs to be changed, is called methylation; a key step in our body's "sanitation."

Now, here's the key to it: Let's say you have a molecule of estrogen and you're done with it, or any other molecule that comes out of your body. It has to be joined up with glutathione (GSH) to be taken out of the body. The GSH takes it to the dump—so to speak—gets rid of it and comes back for another load. If it's a molecule of lead or mercury, or some synthetic thing that your body has never seen before, it puts it in the truck, takes it to the dump, and the truck has to stay at the dump. Now, overloading your detoxification chemistry with this kind of material is very expensive, and it makes for a body that then gets drained by not being able to have enough glutathione to deal with all of this waste. That has an impact that spreads through the whole chemistry. That's where the epidemic of autism can be understood. It's an overload, an excessive total toxic load. Autism is only one of many chronic illnesses that are increasing as a result of environmental toxins.

DB: What are some of the contributors that you think add up over time to this total load theory and lead a child to a state of autism?

SB: I think, broadly speaking, nutrition is one of them; especially a diet too heavy in carbohydrates. Another is antibiotics, which change the composition of the germs that live on, and in, our body and favor the growth of things like fungus, candida, yeast; like the little girl with eczema that I was spoke about earlier. These are things that became familiar to me early on when I met children. Once I saw the first little girl with the yeast problem, then I started looking for more. It turns out there were lots of them. These factors then make children more vulnerable because they have either a high sugar diet or a lot of antibiotics, sometimes only one antibiotic in this little girl's case. This was a classic case. She was a perfectly fine little girl. She had a treatment with antibiotic. She got eczema right afterwards. She had the autism already, but now it went away when we treated with the Nystatin™. In other words, with the antibiotics, the yeast overgrowth had reached some threshold of sensitivity where the eczema revealed the key to her autism. The word sensitivity is one we don't apply to toxins, but that should not be the case. There is an overlap between toxicity and sensitivity.

There are also certain things that we do on purpose to make people sensitive. That is, we want to have a way of warning the body before it encounters certain threats, such as germs, so that a person can respond urgently. It is called immunization. There are two kinds of immunization, one is with live germs and there's another one with dead germs. Let's take the dead ones first. Supposing you have germs called whooping cough (pertussis), and you kill them in a test tube. You then inject them under the skin. The body doesn't care at all about it and doesn't notice it really. It's like getting any other little wound with some dirt in it. This was discouraging to the scientists who were pioneers in the search for ways to immunize us against infectious disease. It turned out that if you mix the dead germs with a certain form of aluminum and inject it, the immune system will say, "Oh my god, this is something bad here." Attention is now drawn to the dead germs and the immune system is forewarned.

The aluminum in this case is called an adjuvant, a term used exclusively for immunizations. The adjuvant says, "Anything nearby is something to remember by way of becoming 'sensitive' to it." What is in the vaccine is not just the dead germs. There are numerous substances that have been used to prepare the dead germs. This may be everything from human protein, egg protein, and other things that go in the processes of making the vaccine. There are some vaccines that contain a little yeast, so you could get sensitized to yeast because it happens to be there with the adjuvant. Do you see what I mean?

The whole question of adjuvants has received attention from an acquaintance of mine, Yehuda Shoenfeld from Israel: one of the world's leading immunologists. In the first few chapters of the book, *Autoimmunity and Immunization,* he says to the world community of scientists in effect, "There's a problem here with adjuvants. We're sensitizing people to things that go way beyond the targeted germ that we're injecting. We must come up with a better adjuvant." Aluminum has been used since long before it's toxicity was recognized. It risks poisoning every child who is immunized, though some are genetically predisposed to be much more sensitive to it than others.

DB: Let's talk a little bit more about the gut, since people outside of our community are just beginning to really understand its importance. Can you talk about the importance of gut health, especially in the context of the prevention of autism?

SB: We've already established that the immune system is a big part of what we're dealing with, the immune system and the brain being one unit that has to do with being sensitive to the world, remembering things and reacting to things. So, it's hard to tease them apart. In medical school, we're taught about these two systems as separate units, but functionally, they are one in the same.

The gut is "outside" us in the sense that it's a tunnel that goes through us. Because this tunnel is permeable, its contents leak into the bloodstream all the time and this then accounts for the burden of detoxification, which is part of the total load we've been speaking about. The gut is full of germs, which also make wonderful things for you. They make vitamins and they do all kinds of really important, vital functions. In fact, recent scientific studies have led researchers to believe that cognitive processes like thinking originate in the gut. It's not unusual in that context to figure that when things go wrong down here [pointing to his gut], then things can go wrong up here [pointing to his brain]. That's what I think is very amply illustrated by all of the people we know who are on the autism spectrum and also in Alzheimer's, Parkinson's, and those who are dealing problems of the aging. It's all one thing.

DB: Can you give parents who might be reading this book a list of some of the triggers that you have heard parents mention that their children experienced prior to being diagnosed with autism?

SB: If I'm giving a lecture and there's a room of two hundred parents there in front of me, and you ask them how many people in the room feel that their child's autism was triggered by a vaccine, "Just raise your hands." Way more than 50 percent of the hands raise instantaneously. I know that the scientific community and various experts keep saying, "It ain't so," but there's lots of good evidence, not just theoretical evidence about the adjuvants and all that, but reputable publications that show that autism can be triggered by immunization, which is sensitizing them and then making them lose tolerance. I think that's the biggest trigger.

Antibiotics are another trigger that may be overlooked by parents and practitioners because they may be less dramatic of an event than getting a bunch of shots in one visit at the doctor. Antibiotics are, moreover, rarely avoided in children these days. We do not know all the factors, such as formula feeding or birth by Caesarian section, that make some children more susceptible to the negative effects of antibiotics.

DB: Tell us why these triggers would have a negative effect just so people could understand. Because when you say vaccines and antibiotics, we think about how great they're supposed to be. I think it's important for parents to understand why, in certain individuals, it becomes a trigger and it's not such a great thing for them.

SB: You're right. The idea that antibiotics can be so mischievous is very disturbing because after all they are great and save a lot of lives. When it comes to antibiotics and children, the number of times that many children get antibiotics is an issue because it becomes a vicious cycle. The first one gets the gut's germs population off-centered because it kills healthy germs in the digestive tract and then the yeast germs are already there. They live in all of us, but they expand their franchise. Now, there are lots of yeast germs and you don't have it necessarily to the point of getting thrush or diaper rash. This makes the immune system crazy because it notices it's too much, and then that makes the immune system more sensitive to lots of things.

And then when the child gets an immunization in the middle of that process, it's even worse. That sequence of events is so commonly found in children. Then people who take issue with this trying to make the connection, "Everybody gets the antibiotics, so how can you tell?" It's true. How can you tell? You would need to do very careful, long-term studies of children to document this. There are certain people in our culture that don't want to do those studies because they don't want to find out these problems that I'm talking about.

C-section is another risk factor because you don't get the flora that a baby is supposed to have of the germs that normally inhabit the vagina, and to some extent from the fecal germs that should cover the baby when its born. A baby born by C-section is deprived of those germs and ends up with different kind of germs in the digestive tract, which don't do the job that the digestive tract germs should be doing for babies—which is to eat the food that comes from the milk and then feed the babies from what they do. In other words, the babies don't digest the milk directly. The baby has the germs work to digest this stuff in the milk and then feed that to the baby. It's a very interesting proposition, and if that was more widely known, people would hesitate to use formula for one thing, and certainly wouldn't hesitate to refrain from doing the proper thing to get the baby inoculated at birth even with C-section. You know the rate of C-section around different parts of world is just staggering, and the babies are paying a big price for that—so that's a risk factor.

DB: Please tell readers how they can inoculate the baby with the necessary good germs at birth in the event they need a C-section?

SB: There is a way to do that, and I've raised some eyebrows when I've re-ferred to it at scientific meetings. I call it the "perineal picnic." I advise putting a finger full of vaginal secretions in the baby's mouth if it's been born by cesarean section. Just that alone, without getting more elaborate in terms of more stuff from the mother's bottom, would be a healthy start. This would be preventive of a lot of problems in babies who are born by C-section. In these cases, since the baby hasn't traveled through the birth canal, it's missing these essential germs. By intro-ducing some of those germs to the baby's mouth—and by extension, gut—some of those germs can start to populate the child's digestive system and stimulate the growth of a normal immune system.

Then, not breastfeeding is another big factor because what's in cow's milk is not the same as what's in mother's milk. Having symptoms of digestive problems early on, having exposure to antibiotics early on, such as the eye drops they place in a baby's eyes, these could be common trig-gers. Think of that, millions of babies are born and they have drops put in their eyes. Now when I was an intern in residency in pediatrics, and I was an attendant in the delivery room, or when I was doing obstetrics, I would say, "Well, I'll put the drops in." If this was a patient that I knew, I knew she didn't have gonorrhea and I would put the drops right here and right here (motioning to each of his own ears). I think this is one of those little things that we do, we don't think about the consequences because this is the way we've always done it. Now that we know more about the sensitivity of the gut flora in the early days of life and the capacity of just enough antibiotics to go in your eye, which of course they go through the tear ducts, down into the nose, then into the digestive system. That's the wrong time to put antibiotics into a baby. All of these things have to do with the health of the gut. This is really where the main story is focused in autism, is the gut. It's where it begins and where it gets complicated in terms of food, feeding, and sensitivities.

DB: When I look back at Dylan's health history and I read it, I cringe because all the signs were there. If you knew the road map to autism, it was perfectly laid out. He had the red cheeks. He had the spit up. It's all there: the drooling, late walking, and late talking. What would you say are some of these signs that someone might see in that first year or two that they should take notice and not say, "Oh, yeah. We'll just keep doing the Miralax™ for eighteen months and that constipation is perfectly fine."

SB: I couldn't agree more with your implication that the digestive tract of an infant is to a great extent subject to abuse by normal doctors. If a child takes antibiotics, then it would be prudent to try to remedy any possible damage to their microbiome. The germs that live in your eyes, nose, mouth all the way down through your digestive track, and on your skin are referred to as the microbiome. Micro meaning small, like the tiny germs, and biome meaning, the living things that are very small and live in your body. When the microbiome gets damaged, it is really hard to fix, but can be done. Sometimes it takes a while, but it means using probiotics and fermented foods that are good for restoring the microbiome, such as lactobacillus and bifidobacterium. It also means a diet that is basically sugar free. Babies shouldn't eat sugar or sweet foods. Staying away from gluten and casein. This seems very extreme to people who have been brought up, as I was, on bread and milk. I mean, it seems unpatriotic to tell people they shouldn't drink milk or eat gluten. But the science thirty years ago and forty years ago when I became involved in this, the evidence was not so strong, but now the evidence is overwhelming that gluten bothers everybody in some way.

Alessio Fasano is the person who first brought this before us. And if he's giving a talk and I'm the moderator, I see the audiences' faces as he's telling people such things as gluten opens the tight junctions, which means that it makes the gut leaky so that things get into the bloodstream that shouldn't be in the bloodstream from the digestive tract. When food goes from the digestive tract into the blood, it must go through a living cell to get to the other side and there it gets inspected, like going through customs. If there are spaces between the cells, it becomes a place where food can get through. That's bad, and gluten opens the tight junctions between the cells in everyone, says Alessio when he's giving his talk. Now he's a professor at Harvard and world famous for coming up with all of this.

When Alessio's giving a talk, he says, "There's only one food that we eat which is gluten that is in wheat, rye, and barley and that's the only food that does this." Germs can make tight junctions open but only one food. Alessio further states, "Gluten opens the tight junctions in everybody," and all the mouths in the audience open wide. When the question and answer comes up and I ask, "Dr. Fasano, you said tight junctions are open in everybody with gluten, but why is it that some people are just fine. They eat pasta and bread and all kinds of wheat things every day and they're fine?" He says, "Well, it's just how long the tight junctions stay open that makes the difference between people in that regard."

Then I say, "Well, if you are worried about proclivity towards some chronic illness that would be of an autoimmune nature by definition, then you should avoid gluten." He says, "Well, yes." I say, "Well, I have this thing called aging which has many of the features of chronic illnesses which includes loss of immune tolerance, so would it be not prudent for me, in order to hedge my bet, to not eat gluten because of that?" He says, "Yes." Now actually when he speaks about this and writes about it, he is quite cautious not to make it sound as if everybody in the world should stop eating gluten. When you're a professor at Harvard, you can't say things like that because the food industry and everybody else would come down on you.

DB: I think what a lot of people don't understand is how toxins can come from the mother. Can you talk a little bit about the mother's body burden? Dr. Nancy O'Hara is going to speak about cleaning up pre-pregnancy, but I just want to touch on the very idea of where else toxins can come from besides the environment so that people understand.

SB: The mother's body is the soil that the baby grows in, and just as in a field of wheat or any other agricultural example, what's in the soil gets into the crop. So, what's in the soil gets into the baby. As it turns out, most of us these days are full of environmental toxins. It's true that we function pretty well with that burden, although it is causing troubles for all of us in some way.

One of my daughters is now twelve weeks pregnant, and she is being so careful about every kind of exposure to anything toxic that you can think of. And rightly so, because the developing organism is so vulnerable to any little thing that could just get a few cells going off in the wrong direction, on the wrong day, and then all of a sudden you've got a problem.

If saying it like that makes people paranoid about it, then they should be paranoid. They should be, if not paranoid, very cautious and not just go buy everything in the supermarket without going organic. The need to eat organic in pregnancy—along with a number of other things that I'm sure you and Nancy will talk about at length are paramount. That certainly is where it all begins.

DB: You talk about how autoimmunity is caused by a loss of tolerance in one's immune system. Can you explain this concept?

SB: I spent a couple of years in Africa as a Peace Corps volunteer in the midst of my residency in pediatrics. For two years, I really didn't see anybody with what you would call an autoimmune problem. Indeed, if I spoke with doctors who'd been there for a long time, like a missionary, about the health of Africans versus the health of the Europeans who were living in Chad, they remarked on how completely different it is. "We never took an appendix out of an African. We never had gall bladder problems." As it happened, they are also really beautiful people, with beautiful teeth and beautiful skin. They didn't have acne, eczema, or allergies of any kind. They wouldn't wheeze with the change of seasons, none of that. Essentially, these were different kinds of human beings health-wise and in many ways better in terms of chronic illnesses.

Of course, as we know from living in countries that are poor because of hygiene and sanitation, the people had more infectious diseases of different kinds and parasites of different kinds, malaria and schistosomiasis and so on. Actually, it turns out that truth be told they were bearing this burden of different organisms like malaria quite well. A group from Johns Hopkins came while I was in Chad and they'd go through a village and draw blood from everybody in the village at noon. Everybody in the village would have malaria parasites in their blood at noon that day, yet they all lined up and they were feeling fine and looking beautiful. Our notion about infectious disease is something that must be reconsidered in this light. Not to romanticize it, but there has to be a little bit of leeway there in terms of what you consider the consequences in an individual of a little malaria. I'm not saying everybody should have malaria. It should be eradicated. It's not a good thing from public health standpoint, but the lesson that I learned there was a lesson that was again in a more scientific way about people over the last thirty or forty years since I was in Chad in the 1960s. That is the people who have these organisms living in their body have something called tolerance, immune tolerance. They are not sensitive in the bad ways we were talking about a few minutes ago.

Tolerance is a treasured feature of any complex system whether it's politics, society, mechanics, or biology. Tolerance is the thing that makes a healthy system or is a representation of its health. Diversity is the other feature. Tolerance and diversity are what makes a healthy complex system. My body is a healthy complex system, so I should be tolerant and I should have diversity in my body especially in terms of all the different kind of germs that live in my body.

Now, I referred to Dr. Schoenfeld from Israel a while ago about his thing, about the adjuvants in vaccines. Dr. Schoenfeld will stand up at a think tank and the first words he says is, "Until proven otherwise, some would say that all chronic illness is autoimmune." And it's true in the sense of when you're dealing with loss of immune tolerance, which is what we're talking about autoimmunity and allergy. Autoimmunity is when you don't tolerate your own thyroid gland or your own skin or some part of you and you're making antibodies to it, or your brain in autism. Children make antibodies against their brain and that's a big part of what's going on in terms of the brain inflammation. He's saying all chronic illness, now he's talking about cancer, cardiovascular disease, diabetes, everything, okay? All chronic illness is autoimmune with very few exceptions, but for practical purposes you have to think about it that way.

DB: When I first came upon this whole autism paradigm, I will never forget that diagram of the three circles overlapping. It showed inflammation, oxidative stress, and then detoxification. Please explain the concept about how all diseases are actually very similar as far as the cause and why people have difficulty comprehending that.

SB: The reason they have a problem with understanding that it's similar is that the medical language is just not suited to learning this different way of thinking. It all comes from the idea that diseases are *things*. Diseases are not things, they are *ideas* that we have about people that have certain things in common. There are unifying features in all chronic illnesses.

They have to do with inflammation, oxidative stress, and problems in detoxification. Those are the three jobs that living things need to take care. When they get damaged, living things get sick.

These three features are common so when I wrote the "Oceanic Disease" paper it was after a meeting in Florida. The theme of the meeting was detoxification, and there were some pretty notable scholars there. I was there talking about autism and I had my diagram, the one that you're referring to. One after the other they would get up and there would be the cancer person, the Parkinson's person, the OBGYN person, and so on. They were all showing the same slides except one person would have a methylation pathway going this way and the other one would have it going this way, but they were all talking about the same things. It was very striking to me because I thought the subject that I was talking about in terms of methylation and all that was in my territory with autism. But this is cancer, heart disease, and everything. They're all looking at the same thing. They've all come to the same conclusion, which is the oceanic disease is the thing that embraces these features that are common to all chronic illness.

Here is a chart that Sid Baker created to illustrate the underlying issues of autism. Note that GSH—glutathione—is a key molecule in all of the three main functions that are common to chronic illness.

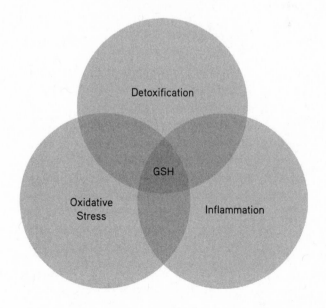

DB: Tell us if you believe that children can recover from autism?

SB: Well, from the 1980s on, I've seen children who would ultimately re-
           cover. The word got around slowly because there was so much resistance
           to the idea. The idea that it was incurable was so fixed in the medical
           mind. Then slowly people began to realize there were children who are
           recovering.

           It's hard to document. I'll give you an example of a boy that I took
           care of who was told by the Yale Child Study Center, which is where I
           saw the film. He was four years old and he was in such bad shape. They
           said, "Look, he's lost. There's no way to get him back. You just should
           put him in an institution because it would be better for his sister not to
           be brought up in a home like this." Now, this was in the 1990s. This is
           the kind of advice that you might have found in the 1960s and you cer-
           tainly wouldn't expect to find it at the Yale Child Study Center, which
           is a pretty advanced, progressive scientific institution, but this is what
           they were told.

           In desperation, that boy's parents heard through the grapevine,
           "You should go see Sid," because I was not far from New Haven and
           Yale, so they came to see me. Long story, but after trying a couple of
           antifungal medicines, it turned out that he had a dramatic response to
           an antifungal medicine, and he got better. We had to stop treatment
           every now and then to see if it was sticking. He would just completely
           fall apart. The people at school didn't know what was going on because
           he'd fallen apart, and then it would take him a few days to get back
           together again when we restarted the medicine. Ultimately, he was able
           to stop taking any antifungals and was no longer autistic. He became
           an artistic prodigy and a chess champion.

           Now, here's the point of my story, why is autism so difficult? After
           he got better, they didn't want to talk about it anymore. This is a nor-
           mal feeling among parents like, "Okay, that was a nightmare in the
           past. We don't want it on his record. We don't want it on his resume.
           He's great now, so let's just be thankful and never mind." That is the
           normal response.

           Then there is the other perspective on the academic side of study-
           ing the differences between children who recover and those who don't,
           which is really an important question. How can that be done if the
           children who have recovered are all in hiding? We don't have the data

to tell us what is it about the children who have recovered comparing them with the ones who haven't, because the difference is so striking. I have children who have recovered rather easily from the steps that we've been talking about. Others where we've just done everything I could think of and has just not worked out.

DB: Can you speak about the children whom you have helped heal and recover from autism? I think it's important to emphasize to parents how children can get better after an autism diagnosis.

SB: They not only get better, but they get to be fabulous people. The vulnerability that children have that is involved in this sensitivity that leads to a loss of tolerance and leads to all of the inflammation, that vulnerability is associated with being sensitive. If it gets to be over the top, then it gets you in trouble. Once you recover, you get to keep those aspects of sensitivity that go along with making you brilliant. The children that I've known who have recovered are just brilliant people. They may keep a few little traits that go with being highly intelligent that we see in people. If you know people that are really, really smart, they sometimes have quirky behaviors and ways about them that are completely socially acceptable. In other words, you still see a little theme that's still in there but it's now embodied in a genius person.

There's a connection between autism and genius as you know. It's a tragedy for our civilization in the sense that I think that the children who are more vulnerable would have been the top ten percent of the smart people. That capacity to be very smart is associated in some way with being sensitive in a way that got them in trouble. So, we're sacrificing not only a generation of children, if we're talking about the ones who don't get better, who don't get treated properly. That is very costly to us as a society because these are precious people.

"There's a connection between autism and genius as you know" is one of my favorite quotes, among many other words of wisdom Dr. Baker shared during our three-hour interview. His words resonate inside me about how precious these children are. Each time I am out in public or on Facebook and I notice another child who has had their life incredibly altered by autism—and not usually for the better. I find it very easy to look at them, seeing past their "autistic features," picturing the life they should be living. It would have been one filled with many friends, a preoccupation with a special hobby, music, or sport they would play. Instead their glorious childhood, the one they should have experienced, gets replaced by a life filled with many painful physical symptoms, daily challenges, and social isolation. Unfortunately, I know about this all too well, as I have endured this journey personally with my beautiful and loving son.

I am hoping that this interview with Dr. Baker and my book can play a small part in shifting the mind-set that we need to take care of our children before they develop a chronic illness or disease. Many of us are well-aware of how toxic our environment has become, and it is time to be proactive and do everything we can to prevent illness before it occurs. Remember the world is always changing and it is not the same as when you or I grew up.

I purposely chose to put this interview first, as Dr. Baker touches on many different subjects that may be novel concepts to you right now. Each one of these new approaches toward looking at chronic illness and its prevention will be broken down further and discussed in greater detail in each of the subsequent chapters. This interview can be reflected on as an important overview to the many areas there are to make changes and adopt a healthier lifestyle, such as altering one's diet, questioning certain medical practices even though they have always been around, and making careful decisions that ultimately determine which toxins you are exposed to.

One of the most useful concepts that Dr. Baker is famous for talking about is that every disease is caused by the same underlying factors, which is illustrated in that chart on page 47. The meaning I hope you take away from this umbrella of diseases concept, which he explains in his story about the conference with the famous scholars, is that each one of us should do all the same things for ourselves that are outlined in this book. I know the point of picking up this book is to prevent autism in your child. However, if adopting a healthier lifestyle can lower your child's risk of developing a debilitating chronic illness such as autism, then wouldn't it make sense that it could help you from developing one too?

I currently practice a lot of healthy habits each day to keep myself feeling good and to prevent a chronic illness from developing. There is no one specific disease that I am concerned with, like some people who have a history of a specific type of cancer that runs in the family. Sure, I have a ton of dementia and Alzheimer's in my family, but who knows how my specific genes will get expressed in my lifetime. It could be cancer or some other dreaded illness that wasn't so common during the time when my ancestors were alive. For this reason, it is of extreme importance that you try to look at the whole picture just as these functional medicine practitioners view the body as a whole. You cannot just adjust one small area of your diet for instance and expect the results to be miraculous. Keeping oneself healthy takes a lot of effort in a bunch of different areas, but I promise you the results will be so rewarding that you won't even consider it work after a while, but a mere change in your lifestyle. I try to eat the majority of my meals at home, made from organic unprocessed ingredients, supplement with specific nutrients I feel my body needs and this is always changing. And lastly staying away from toxic compounds is of great importance as I feel that my family is particularly vulnerable, since our individual chemistry does not allow us to detox so easily. For me, this has just become a new way of life that is necessary to feel good and be healthy. I no longer view this as an arduous task that has to be done. I am forty-five years old and feel better than I did in my twenties. Back then I was plagued with anxiety, poor memory and concentration, skin issues, subpar energy, and an overall feeling of malaise. It took a lot of work to get where I am now and I wouldn't trade it for anything in the world.

CHAPTER SUMMARY

Autism is a result of a loss of immune tolerance.

The total load theory is when the body gets overwhelmed with too many toxins and is not able to work properly and detoxify itself. These toxins can build up and overwhelm an overtaxed immune system, causing the body to become quite ill. The people most at risk are the very young and old.

Some common contributing factors for autism are a diet that is too high in sugar or carbohydrates, too many antibiotics, and vaccines.

Gut health is very important. It plays a role in important functions such as making vitamins and our thinking.

C-section is one risk factor that puts a baby at higher risk for autism, since the baby does not inherit the proper gut flora from its mother during the birth process.

A baby can be inoculated with the proper germs in the event that the mother needs to have a C-section.

Gluten opens the tight junctions in the gut and allows things to make their way into the bloodstream where they don't belong. How long they stay open depends on the individual.

All diseases have the same three underlying causes: inflammation, oxidative stress, and detoxification issues.

Children can recover from autism.

CHAPTER 5

PRECONCEPTION & PREGNANCY PREVENTION FOR AUTISM

With Nancy Hofreuter O'Hara, MD

Dr. Nancy O'Hara first planted the seed in my head many years ago that I could change the course of autism in my next child, starting long before I got pregnant. So, I took this gift that she gave me and ran miles with it until I could run no more. I believe it was this early verbal intervention during one of my son's first few visits to her office that helped me to prevent my daughter from getting autism. Nancy will always have my gratitude for this, and for sharing all the valuable information from the following interview with all of you.

Dr. O'Hara is an extremely passionate individual who not only takes care of adults and children with complex chronic illness, but she also works tirelessly to train other physicians on how to treat and prevent chronic illness in their patients as well. She graciously gives her time in interviews for books and films on the subject. Her interest in doing so is to spread the information far and wide that we need not suffer with chronic illness, and the more important message is that we have the ability to prevent and heal from one as well. She's dedicated her life to alleviating the suffering of countless people.

Dr. Nancy O'Hara first began her work with special needs children as a teacher. Then she went on to earn a medical degree from the University of Pennsylvania and completed her residency and chief residency at The University of Pittsburgh. Dr. O'Hara's practice focuses on an integrative approach to treat children that have neurodevelopmental disorders such as autism, ADHD, PANDAS (Pediatric Autoimmune Neuropsychiatric Disorders Associated with Strep), and Lyme.

I am extremely excited about the information that you are about to gain in this next chapter, since I know it will make a dramatic difference for you and your child.

DB: I always find that in order to do something about a problem, we first have to realize that there is a problem. So the first question I'm going to ask you is whether you think autism is increasing?

NHO: Absolutely. The rates of autism have skyrocketed—thirty years ago, I was teaching children with autism and it was one in ten thousand. It's now one in twenty-seven boys in the state of New Jersey, one in sixty-eight overall. That's a huge increase. The answer can't be that we as physicians are just diagnosing better. This is a clinical diagnosis. My parents' and our grandparents' generation were good diagnosticians. There is no way that better diagnosis alone has brought about this astronomical increase.

DB: Would you call the proportions of the increase an epidemic?

NHO: Definitely.

DB: Do you think children are sicker today than they were ten years ago?

NHO: Yes. We are raising a generation of children to be three things: 1) vitamin D deficient; 2) iodine deficient; and 3) biome depleted. Our biomes, our ecosystems are deficient in the plethora of germs that allow us to be healthy, and that's a very important reason why all of our kids are weaker, generationally and individually, than our generation and our parents' generation.

DB: Do you think autism can be prevented?

NHO: Autism can be prevented, not in a hundred percent of the cases. There is a genetic predisposition, but there are definitely environmental triggers, and if we can look at what those triggers are and remove those triggers, either prenatally—or immediately postnatally—then we can make a big impact on the number of children with autism.

DB: I'm going to talk about how you were one of the first practitioners nine years ago to talk to me about cleaning out. Can you speak to this concept of cleaning out before you get pregnant, and the benefits it provides to both the mother and her unborn child?

NHO: We, as moms, not only pass on our genes, but we pass on our germs. We pass on all of the things within our bodies to our children. We as the vessel for our children have to be clean, that means gastrointestinally, immunologically, and metabolically. Mothers have to be as healthy as we can be before we get pregnant. Individually what that means is we have to make sure that our guts are clean and that we're having one stool a day, we don't have an overgrowth of germs such as yeast in particular, and that we are eating a good, anti-inflammatory diet. As my friend Stu Freedenfeld says, "There's no such thing as junk food. It's either junk or it's food," and if we eat foods without barcodes then we are being healthier. Then we need to make sure our immune systems are healthy, that we do not have things in our systems, vaccines and the components and additives in them that may alter our immune systems directly before we get pregnant—or certainly while we're pregnant.

Next we have to detoxify our environments. Our makeup, does it have lead in it? Our ceramics and the products within our home, do they have other heavy metals that can cause problems? Our homes themselves, are they full of mold or metals, chemicals or other toxins that may be problematic? Then it's about asking very simple things like, what's in what we're eating every day? Is our diet as organic as possible? All of those things are very important in keeping us healthy and therefore making us more likely to have healthy children.

DB: When do you suggest that a woman would start this cleanout process?

NHO: I would start the cleanout process when you're a teenager, but that's very hard to do. Certainly as a young woman, the more you can take care of your body, the better. At the very least it has to be three months before you get pregnant, but it would be much better if it were at least a year before, because there are mineral levels, vitamin levels, as well as levels of germs and toxins you have to monitor, which may take quite a while before you get pregnant.

DB: Let's talk a little bit about the cleanout process in greater detail, just so people have a general idea of what that would entail, of course, recognizing that it's going to be different for each individual. Tell us a little bit about implementing this concept?

NHO: So initially you need to look at your home and you need to measure your home, both the water and the soil outside your home and anything that you use all the time, like your bedding, your tub, or shower and measure those for chemicals and metals that could be toxic. We spend a third of our life in bed, organic mattresses, organic and one-hundred percent cotton sheets, and allergenic covers are very important. That would be the first step, and then getting rid of any of those that are problematic.

The second step in that metal and chemical testing would be to test ourselves, to see if we have any burdens of those metals, chemicals, or toxins in our systems and remove those as naturally as possible. This may just be through natural detoxification, homeopathic detoxification, sauna, extra amounts of glutathione and N-acetylcysteine, things that would detoxify us.

Then we need to look at our gastrointestinal systems. Are we constipated? Anybody that's not pooping at least once a day and up to three times a day is constipated. Doesn't have to be the little hard rabbit pellets, it can be a normal stool, but only every other day. So making sure we're not constipated and taking extra magnesium, aloe, vitamin C, fluids, and fiber to ensure that. Checking ourselves for signs of germ overgrowth, particularly yeast. I always say anybody who acts "drunk" in any way may well be yeasty. That can be a person with brain fog. It can be a person with inappropriate laughter or giggling, a person that's more combative than normal, or experiencing severe PMS can certainly be a sign of yeast overgrowth. We can safely rid our bodies of that overgrowth with high doses of probiotics, Saccharomyces Boulardii, which is a prebiotic, and sometimes antifungal herbs or medications.

Then I think we need to look at ourselves immunologically. A lot of us have underlying autoimmune diseases, and that's where the immune system is attacking itself—it can be thyroiditis, migraine headaches, lupus, or diabetes.

We need to carefully examine whether we have any evidence of inflammation and autoimmune disease, and treat that appropriately by decreasing that inflammation prior to getting pregnant.

DB: Let's talk a little bit about the fact that a lot of women who go on to have a baby may suffer from allergies. Please explain how having allergies or an autoimmune disease can be a risk factor?

NHO: Several ways—when a person has allergies, or what's called atopic disease, there's a shift in our T cells. We have more T cells fighting allergies rather than fighting infections, and that is something we can genetically, as well as immunologically, pass on to our children. In addition to that, there are antibodies or proteins within the moms that can cross the blood brain barrier and affect the developing fetus.

DB: Could something as simple as food allergies that are undetected affect the baby if the mother keeps eating that food during pregnancy and creates that negative immune response?

NHO: Sure. We know when a mom is breastfeeding if the baby has diarrhea or develops a rash; it may well be from something that the mom is eating. If the mom removes milk for instance from her diet and the rash or the diarrhea goes away, then that means that the baby may well be sensitive to it. That same thing may be going on when we're pregnant, and that sensitivity or allergic response that we have to a food (that we may think is very minor) may well be passed on immunologically into our developing fetus.

DB: Could you explain to people the significance of the mother's body burden especially as it relates during pregnancy to the developing child?

NHO: We live in a toxic world, so we are all burdened by exposure to metals: aluminum, mercury, lead, cadmium, fluoride, even within our bodies, but much of that crosses the placenta and gets into our children when we're pregnant. So if we have high levels of any of those metals, as well as chemicals, organophosphates, pesticides, etc., those can cross the placenta and get into our fetus. The developing fetus is much less able to handle those amounts of chemicals and metals than grown adults are. Just think about basic surface area, plus the developing brain. They are unable to handle that burden that we may not even feel, but they may have tremendous negative consequences from it.

DB: How can a mother test herself to see if she has an accumulation of heavy metals?

NHO: The first way is to check your home. You can go to Lowe's or Home

Depot and get a home check for lead as well as other metals, and you can check your bathtub, water, and soil. You can also employ a home inspector to do all those things, as you would if you bought a new home.

Secondly, you can check your own levels within your hair, which is a very easy one to do. This will tell you your exposure to those metals within the last three months. You can also check your urine, which will tell you within the last couple of weeks your exposure to those metals.

If it's something you're very concerned about because you're a dental hygienist or dentist and you have large exposures to mercury, or you work in a plant, you've been a smoker—you can go to a physician or practitioner and have those levels checked in your blood, in your urine, and perhaps even do a provocative challenge before you get pregnant to see if your levels are high and then to work on removing them.

Consider mercury for example. Several of our vaccines that we still get when we're pregnant have mercury in them, like several of our flu vaccines. As far as amalgams, there are studies that show that a mother who has had greater than six silver fillings have a higher likelihood of having a child with autism. And certainly fish consumption, any large fish, particularly from the Atlantic Ocean area can contain high levels of mercury. Looking at all of those things as you're looking at your history is very important.

DB: Is there a safe way for women to deal with amalgams before they're pregnant such as seeing a special dentist?

NHO: Yes. If you're going to remove your amalgams and replace them with composite fillings, you need to do it safely. Every time you chew, for every amalgam in your mouth, you're releasing thirteen micrograms of mercury every day and that's getting into your fetus. If you remove those unsafely, you are absorbing all of that mercury you're trying to take out. You have to do it safely, you have to do it with extra vitamin C and you can go online and find dentists that do this correctly, so that it's not a risk to you or your potential child.

DB: Now let's talk about nutrition during pregnancy, because a lot of women use that time as, "Oh I'm going to gain the forty, fifty pounds anyway, I might as well enjoy myself." Let's talk about why monitoring what you eat is so important during pregnancy?

NHO: Nutrition is the fuel for our body. Nutrition is important for all of us every day, but especially when we're eating for your unborn child it is that much more important. The best way to decrease inflammation, which is the common denominator in what goes wrong for many of our children is by decreasing inflammation in our diets. An anti-inflammatory diet is a diet that's high in fresh vegetables, fresh fruits, and proteins. Some good organic meats, nuts, seeds, beans, and low in sugars, definitely low in junk food and low in complex carbohydrates, which we often think of as our comfort foods. I think we need to find other comfort foods when we're pregnant that may be healthier for our children, a good spaghetti squash for instance rather than a bowl of pasta.

DB: What types of things should women think about trying to limit or avoid during pregnancy?

NHO: Well first with regard to food, I think the more organically you can eat, the better, especially avoiding what used to be called the "dirty dozen" which is now the top fifteen most problematic foods, and again you can find that online. I think secondly anything that is a processed food and has multiple lines of what's in it can be problematic and inflammatory. I think the organic foods are most important. Secondly, I think smoking and alcohol need to be avoided, as well as staying in environments with high levels of secondhand smoke.

Thirdly, look at where you work. You're spending a lot of time there, are there any chemical exposures there? Any time you lay down a new carpet or buy a new piece of furniture or paint, you are being exposed to new chemicals. All of those things need to be what's called outgassed for several days, which means putting them outside, opening them up and allowing the chemicals to not be in your living room and in any enclosed space initially. Dry cleaning is another one that a lot of chemicals are contained especially when you bring them home and leave them in the plastic. Unwrap those, leave them out for a while, before you put them away in your closet.

So those are very simple measures, and there are amazing websites where you can go to find all this information, like the Environmental Working Group, EWG.org, will have a lot of information on these exposures you need to avoid.

DB: Let's discuss some other things that people don't normally talk about, which is the birth process. What are your thoughts about minimizing risks during the birth process?

NHO: I think the first thing to remember is that stress in any way is the greatest contributor to an increase in inflammation. Any way that you can decrease your stress and make the birth process easier on you, will also make it easier on the baby; seek out a warm environment, an environment filled with music that you enjoy, with lighting that makes you feel better, with pillows or a person that helps to relieve your stress is very important. There have been a couple of studies that showed an increased incidence of autism with the use of Pitocin, which is a medication that's used to induce birth. There have not been any other studies that have shown any of the other chemicals that we use can be problematic, but again, the less the better. The less things that you can use to have a more natural vaginal birth, the better.

DB: Now let's talk about why having an elective C-section may not be best for your baby. Obviously if you have to have one for medical reasons, then there's nothing to even think about. However, if you're scheduling one because you want your doctor or you want it on a certain day, please let people know why this is not the greatest idea?

NHO: As I said, as moms we give our genes but also our germs to our children. The germs that are most beneficial for our infants are the germs that come through the vaginal process. When we have a child born by C-section, they are missing those germs. They have a much greater risk of abnormal germs, by having increased yeast, but also less bacteroides and increased firmicutes. These are germs that we don't want our babies to have. Their guts are filled with our skin germs rather than our vaginal germs, and that can be very problematic for their growth later.

What's very important in all of our children I think, but especially those born by C-section, is to give probiotics from the beginning, and those are normal germs. You have to give a good probiotic that is high in billions of flora and give that to ourselves if we're breastfeeding and to our babies when we stop breastfeeding or if we're not.

DB: Is there anything else that they can do if they have to have a C-section to try to build up the baby's gut flora? A probiotic is of course one thing that they can speak to their pediatrician about.

NHO: Certainly breastfeeding after birth, even if you can only do it for a few days to a few weeks. That baby needs your colostrum, which is the first milk, the highest immunogenic milk that our babies need for good immune function. Even if your baby is born prematurely or doesn't have a good suck and swallow for different reasons, pumping and giving that breast milk would be of utmost importance.

DB: What are some options for those women who cannot breastfeed? I was one of those people that tried really hard and it just didn't work out as I planned. So I did the Weston A. Price Foundation homemade baby formula. Can you tell people what options they can explore with their pediatrician?

NHO: Sure. Certainly the Weston Price homemade baby formula is one of the best. If you can't do that for varied reasons, looking at other formulas that are more elemental, more easily digested may be something to do. In addition to that, adding essential fatty acids. Essential fatty acids are just that, essential to our development, and we get a lot of essential fatty acids, particularly DHA from breast milk. But If we're not getting breast milk, than formula is probably not enough and not in the right proportions for our baby, so giving an additional essential fatty acid, a small amount of cod liver oil, or DHA to EPA ratio from one of the trusted essential fatty acid brands would be advised.

DB: What are some supplements that a mother should keep in mind to talk to her OB about or consider taking? Could you tell us some things that you think are important?

NHO: The two most essential, as I have said, are probiotics and essential fatty acids. Then vitamin D would be the next because most of us are deficient in vitamin D. We live indoors more and we're wearing sunscreen all the time when we're outside. We're not getting the sunlight exposure that we need. So we need vitamin D and our babies need it, especially in breast-fed babies often they need it more than even formula-fed babies. Then I think if there were one test that I would love to be added to the infant heel prick, it would be a measure of glutathione. Glutathione is the mother lode molecule of all of our bodies. It's what we all need to detoxify, to get these chemicals, metals, toxins, allergens, and germs, out of our systems.

What we know is that children with autism have a seventy-one to seventy-two percent decrease in reduced or good glutathione (GSH). And instead they have oxidized glutathione. Good glutathione looks like this with a sulfur molecule sticking off of it, so think of it as being sticky and sticking to those things we want to get out of our system. What our kids with autism have is a lot more of GSSG (glutathione disulfide), where the two sticky molecules are stuck together. Well if your sticky parts are stuck together, they can't effectively stick to and get out of the system those chemicals and toxins.

So if we knew early on that a baby had a low level of glutathione, we could give them that either through N-acetylcysteine or glutathione, or the components that make up glutathione, supplementing B12 or folinic acid or zinc or other B vitamins that they may need to help produce glutathione, which may be helping to prevent what we now know as autism.

DB: How easy is it to test glutathione levels? And how could people go about getting one?

NHO: It's a very easy blood test, very inexpensive, and you can get it at any time. You do need to make sure what you're measuring though because if you measure a total glutathione, you will get a combination of reduced and oxidized, good and bad respectively. You could have seventy percent good and thirty percent bad and it'll look the same as seventy percent bad, thirty percent good. You need to make sure you're getting either a cysteine level, which is the first layer before glutathione, or getting a reduced glutathione level and measure that, but it's very easy to do.

In addition to the glutathione, what you can measure through a regular lab test is a genetic defect called MTHFR (methylenetetrahydrofolate reductase), which we fondly call the mother (whispers profanity) gene, because it really messes up your folate metabolism. And because that's very important in making glutathione, it can really mess up your glutathione metabolism as well. A simple blood test or a buccal swab is all it takes. It's available in at-home buccal swabs for genetic testing, and that one is very important.

The other thing you can get through a regular lab test is what's called a homocysteine level, which is something that we measure for people with heart disease. Our children with autism can also have very abnormal homocysteine levels, and that can be an indicator that this pathway of methylation and sulfation making glutathione can be abnormal.

DB: What is the importance of MTHFR? Why is it a good idea to measure it, and how would it increase the risk?

NHO: Let me first explain folate metabolism. Folate is a B vitamin that we get in our diets, mainly through green leafy vegetables, which our kids aren't getting much of anyway but they should. That gets broken down to folinic acid. Folinic acid is what pregnant mothers take to prevent neural tube defects, Spina Bifida, and that's what's in maternal multivitamins and prenatal vitamins, then that gets broken down to methly tetrahydrofolate. Methyltetrahydrofolate is what we really need for this glutathione pathway and what we need for our brains. That's what gets into our brains to prevent what's called cerebral folate deficiency in the brain. This deficiency causes brain fog, cognitive delays, and anxiety, so we really need enough folate into our brains.

When we have this genetic defect of MTHFR, we have a block at a fork in the road. We can't take the folate from our foods and make it into the methyltetrahydrofolate that we need for our brains and that we need for glutathione production. If we know we have that defect, then we need to give as a supplement either folinic acid or methyltetrahydrofolate to better serve our brains and our metabolism.

DB: What does this pathway do? What's the biggest thing it helps our body do?

NHO: Folation in general is important for several reasons. First, it's a very calming supplement or product within our food. It decreases anxiety, agitation, tics, and obsessive compulsive disorder. Second, folation is part of the pathway of glutathione production. Folation and methylation are the upper parts of a pathway of glutathione production. Third, folate in the methylfolate gets through the blood brain barrier and into our brain to help brain function, mainly cognitive function. Without it we have developmental delays and brain fog.

DB: Is this because this pathway helps with detoxification?

NHO: Yes, glutathione is the major detoxifier in our body and folation is one of the first parts of making glutathione and of natural detoxification in our bodies.

DB: Is a woman able to take regular folic acid if she is positive for this MTHFR? Is that the best source for her?

NHO: Folic acid is folate, and if she has the MTHFR defect, that's not the best source. She wants to look at something that's called folinic acid, the brand name that you can get as a prescription is Leucovorin™ and many pregnant mothers take that or methyltetrahydrofolate. Those are the two metabolites or breakdown products of folate or folic acid that you need to take if you have an MTHFR defect.

DB: Does the MTHFR defect put a child at an increased risk of autism?

NHO: There's been no proof that it puts a child at increased risk, but eighty percent of children with autism have an MTHFR defect, whereas it's more like twenty percent in the general population. So there's a co-incident perhaps or causative relationship, it's never been proven scientifically though. But again, remembering that methylfolate, that metabolite of folate is very important in our glutathione production and there has been a causative relationship between low glutathione and autism.

DB: Tell us about the significance of the cerebral folate autoantibody. This is something of course you know came back positive for my daughter.

NHO: There are antibodies that can be produced in your brain called cerebral folate antibodies. What they do is they block the entrance of methyl tetrahydrofolate into the brain, so that derivative of folate that you need to drive your brain function is blocked at the blood brain barrier. You can test for that in a blood test, and if you have that particular antibody, then you can flood the system so to speak with much higher doses of folinic acid or methyltetrahydrofolate to get more of what's needed into the brain and to decrease the symptoms of cerebral folate deficiency, which again are brain fog, cognitive delays, anxiety, agitation, sometimes lethargy, and you can decrease those by giving high doses, mega doses of folinic acid or methyltetrahydrofolate.

DB: What are the best things that a mother who already has a child on the spectrum can do to try to prevent it in her next child? Is there anything extra that she needs to do after the baby is born?

NHO: I think an anti-inflammatory diet, an organic diet, probiotics, essential fatty acids, and possibly getting the child tested for these things we're talking about. Getting an MTHFR blood test. If you know your other child, for instance, has cerebral folate deficiency, measuring that, and measuring levels of inflammation. Simple measures like a C-reactive protein or a sed rate or an antinuclear antibody, and treating for inflammation if it is there. Looking for evidence of yeast, a child that's born and certainly has evidence of thrush or a yeast diaper rash or seborrheic dermatitis they may need much higher doses of probiotics or the mother may need to take antifungal herbs while she's breastfeeding.

Those are all things we need to look at, and then mineral deficiencies, vitamin deficiencies, vitamin D as we've said, but some of these children are deficient in vitamin A. Some of them are deficient in vitamin C. Those are very essential antioxidants. Some are deficient in minerals like zinc, selenium, iron, and those are things that may well need to be looked at.

DB: Let's talk about some of the soft signs, which are what functional medicine practitioners refer to as the early warning signs. Many of these are considered very normal by regular doctors such as constipation, food sensitivities, and constant ear infections just to name a few. Why is it important to take note of these seemingly benign symptoms especially if we're seeing a lot of them?

NHO: The first, very early in the neonatal period, may be hyperbilirubinemia, which is jaundice. A child that has jaundice without an ABO incompatibility with mom, without excessive dehydration may be showing that they're having problems with conjugation, and that may be an early sign that they have problems again in that metabolism, possibly that glutathione pathway. It has been shown that kids with high bilirubinemias are more likely to have autism later in life. That's the first thing.

The second thing would be prolonged or out of the ordinary colic. A child that is hyper irritable not just at the end of the day but earlier in the day or for prolonged periods of time may be showing you that they have more gastrointestinal distress. A child that has excessive reflux may well have yeast overgrowth or small intestinal bacterial overgrowth rather than just positional reflux. That's something to look at. Those are the most important ones, and then the next would be lack of reciprocity, lack of looking and smiling at a person, fixating on objects rather than the person. These would be very early signs that we need to intervene.

DB: What about some of the ones that you might see a little bit later like food allergies, eczema, and constipation? What do these signs mean for the children that have to take Miralax™ for a long period of time or are constantly on antibiotics?

NHO: Well first, constipation may be a sign again of gastrointestinal abnormalities. If a child has germ overgrowth, dysbiosis, the germs are loving life. They're in a warm, moist environment and they want to stay there. That may be one of the reasons that the child has constipation. Treating that constipation naturally is very important. Remembering again, constipation is any child that's not pooping at least once a day. Using things like magnesium, particularly magnesium citrate in a constipated child, vitamin C, aloe in a very good form. Remembering aloe needs to be certified. Those are very important in treating a child with constipation.

Then reflux, again, rather than putting Prevacid™ or Prilosec™ or some medication to suppress the symptoms, looking at why a child may have reflux. Usually again, it's because of germ overgrowth, GI (gastrointestinal) distress and inflammation due to an abnormal amount of germs. Probiotics, a good diet, and all those things that I mentioned to treat that may be very helpful.

Then we go to the child with allergies, eczema, atopic dermatitis, or food allergies in particular, these are early signs that the child may have an immunologic disregulation. Their immune system may be hyperstimulated, overstimulated, again by germ overgrowth, or they may have antibodies from their moms that cause them to be more hyperstimulated. Again, we would need to look at that and decrease the overstimulation, with the same things again, treating the germs, probiotics, essential fatty acids, and an anti-inflammatoryaloe, BH4, curcumin all decrease that inflammation rather than just lathering with hydrocortisone or using steroids.

DB: Just to drive the point home to people who have not had a child on the spectrum. Can these little things keep snowballing into something more serious? Can you explain that briefly?

NHO: Absolutely. All of these things we're talking about are triggers, and one trigger may just be one simple problem, but when you put one trigger on top of another trigger on top of another trigger that's on top of genetic predisposition, then you may end up with a much more severely affected child with a severe atopic problem, a severe autoimmune problem, or a severe neurodevelopmental problem like autism. When you have a child with reflux, constipation, frequent ear infections, atopic dermatitis, or eczema, with other allergies, those may all come together to then both make that child more susceptible to further problems but also be a clue that from the get-go they were susceptible and we need to do more to prevent further problems and not just treat the present ones.

DB: Have you seen other children, aside from Jessica, whose parents holistically treated the eczema, and each of these other issues that were coming up? And did they have a successful outcome of preventing autism or other chronic illnesses?

NHO: We've had hundreds within our practice and two of my colleagues have actually written papers. I have a consultative practice, so I am seeing people a little bit later down the line. Two of my colleagues that have primary care practices in instituting these things early on, treating allergic conditions and constipation and reflux naturally, giving probiotics and essential fatty acids from the get-go and spreading out vaccines. They are treating ear infections more naturally with garlic and mullein oil or herbs. In doing that, they have markedly reduced and written articles about this reduction in the incidence of autism.

DB: What are some of these contributors that you think add up? In Dylan's case, I have a very long list. When you look back at some of these health histories, whether it's autism or asthma, what are some of the main contributors that you see?

NHO: We have a thirty-page questionnaire that we have everybody fill out, so we're getting the entire history. First, a family history, particularly a maternal history of autoimmune disease, that's number one. Secondly then, what are the maternal exposures before the baby is born? What medications did they have? What stressors do they have? Then looking at the immediate natal and prenatal period. What medications did the baby get? What vaccines did the baby get? What antibiotics did the baby get? Then going on the neonatal period, is the baby born by C-section? Was the baby breastfed? Does the baby have repeated infections? Does the baby have repeated evidence of yeast? Again, thrush, yeast diaper rash, and seborrheic dermatitis? Does the baby have an allergic condition, either skin or food allergies or environmental sensitivities.

Then we look at what are the exposures within the home. Have there been tick exposures, as in Lyme disease? Have there been mold exposures as in water? What are the electromagnetic fields around the house? What are the metal exposures and chemical exposures? All of those add up and it's not that any one of them is the sole trigger. We're always looking for the sound bite. This causes autism. It's not that I'm saying that any one of those cause autism, but it's a tipping point. It's the straw that breaks the camel's back. It's the last little drop of water in the bucket that makes it overflow.

DB: What is autism?

NHO: Well first autism is a label. It's just a word that we've put on a child that has problems with communication, problems with perseverative behaviors, and problems with social and emotional communication. However, what we really look at is what's going on deeper than that. What are the gastroenterologic, the gut, the immunologic, and the metabolic conditions that may be going wrong in an individual child that may lead them to show the outward signs of this label.

DB: Do you consider autism to be an autoimmune illness?

NHO: Yes. That's the immunologic piece. The immune system is dysregulated. The proteins or antibodies are in many cases attacking the brain and causing inflammation within the brain.

DB: Let's talk about a huge issue going on today with women not being able to conceive. What does it mean when a woman cannot procreate? It seems like we have an epidemic of women who cannot get pregnant and have no choice but to try IVF, which sometimes does not even work for them. Many of these women are needing surrogates because they can't get pregnant even after many rounds of IVF. Tell us what that's all about.

NHO: I think that our human body is meant to have children, but if we are toxic, if we are ill, if we have an autoimmune disease, that may be a sign that our body is saying I'm not well enough, I'm not healthy enough to make another human being. I think we need to look at our own health before again we just put a medicine on it and force a pregnancy. I speak from that personally because I certainly had difficulty getting pregnant, and I think what I found for myself is that I had tremendous yeast overgrowth. I was tremendously toxic and needed to detoxify. I had several mineral and vitamin deficiencies, and I had several blocks energetically in different ways that needed to be cleared. In doing that I was able then to get pregnant. Those are all things we all need to look at in ourselves to help be as healthy as we can, to then have a healthy baby more naturally.

DB: We use the word epidemic softly, but there is somewhat of an epidemic of thyroid issues, especially with women, and there's been a lot of talk about how that can be a big contributor to having a child with autism. Can you tell me about that and if you think a woman should simply just get tested before or during the pregnancy to find out about that?

NHO: Ideally, I think all women should get tested for inflammation and autoimmune disease, thyroid being the most common but diabetes is another, inflammatory bowel disease is another, any autoimmune condition will increase your risk of having a child with an autoimmune condition.

I think more than anything else in today's society we have depleted our biomes, our ecosystems of the plethora of germs that we need. And in that biome depletion, which used to be called the hygiene hypothesis, we have seen a great increase in autoimmune diseases. We didn't see these in pre-industrialized society. We didn't see thyroiditis, autoimmune disease, inflammatory bowel disease, diabetes, autism, and ADHD, and all of these diseases in pre-industrialized society. Part of the reason for that may well be that we have depleted our ecosystems of the plethora of germs that we need, and that's not just antibiotics and antibacterial soaps. That's wearing shoes, using toilets, living indoors more with less vitamin D exposure, C-sections, not breastfeeding. All of those lead to the depletion of our biomes and the increase in autoimmune disease in moms as well as our babies.

DB: Is prevention multifaceted? It seems that the world is so toxic today that you can't just do one thing and expect to have your risks completely minimized. Can you talk about how you might need to do several things simultaneously?

NHO: Everything is multifaceted, the cause of these diseases as well as the prevention of them. We need to look at number one, our stress. Anything that increases stress externally, emotional, psychological stress, will increase stress physiologically. When we're stressed, we're more acidic. When we're more acidic, think of things as being rusty. When we're rusty, we don't work as well. None of our internal processes are going to work as well if we're stressed. One way to prevent is to decrease stress. However you do that, it may be by going for a run, doing yoga, listening to music or meditation, whatever it is, decreasing stress.

The second thing is to make our guts, our gastrointestinal systems as healthy as possible. That's by eating good diets, taking probiotics, and decreasing inflammation. The third is decreasing inflammation overall, providing a good healthy immune system, by treating any autoimmune disease like thyroiditis that we may have and decreasing our inflammation overall. Then fourth would be our metabolism and supporting our metabolism, which again is mostly by a good anti-inflammatory diet, but making sure we have the vitamins and minerals that we need. The antioxidants like vitamin C, A, D, and E, as well as the minerals that we need to make our detoxification systems work as well as they should.

DB: We always go back to the gut all the time. Please explain this for people who have nothing to do with autism and don't have a child on the spectrum. Why is the gut so important?

NHO: The gut's the second brain. In my opinion, it may be the first brain. All of the things that we talk about in our brains: serotonin, dopamine, norepinephrine, epinephrine actually are in the gut. Seventy percent of our immune system starts in the gut. The first line of defense, secretory IgA, which is an immunoglobulin that is meant to defend us from all outside triggers is in the gut. Where do we get our fuel? Through our gut. If we're not putting high-octane fuel into our machinery, then we may get a lot more knocks and pings, just like our cars. We need to put the best fuel in to get the best energy and result out.

DB: Now you're a doctor who uses a lot of natural herbs, special diets, and pharmaceutical interventions when it's necessary. The average person is so used to going to the pharmacy every time something's wrong and picking up a prescription. Do you think there are some easy ways to treat these everyday minor ailments more holistically?

NHO: There are for almost all pharmaceutical, especially over the counter, interventions to treat something, there are natural ways to treat it. There are a plethora of them. We talked about someone with constipation using magnesium, vitamin C, and aloe rather than Miralax™. For ear infections, garlic and mullein oil drops and anti-analgesics rather than immediately going to antibiotics. For reflux: aloe, licorice, slippery elm, marshmallow, digestive enzymes. For atopic dermatitis or eczema: again using an anti-inflammatory, like essential fatty acids and aloe and natural emulients like shea butter, and all of those things to treat naturally.

DB: Is there anything that you wish would change in the medical paradigm with preventing and treating autism specifically?

NHO: First of all, my mentor always taught me if you listen they will come. I think the first thing we need to do as physicians is to listen. If we really spend time listening to our families, we will learn a lot more about how to take care of these children and about how to prevent autism or catch autism much earlier on. I think the second thing is adding that glutathione to the infant heel prick and looking for the children that may be more at risk. Then I think the last thing would be to individualize medicine as much as possible. It is not one size fits all. We can have standard of care without making every child do the exact same thing at the exact same time.

We may have to individualize our ear infection protocol, diet protocol, or our vaccine protocol for an individual that may be more at risk. We need to be open to looking at families that have the greatest peril of having a child with autism.

I think there are a subset of children that have vaccine injuries, and I'm not sure if it's actually the vaccine but the vehicle with which it is placed. So it may be aluminum or formaldehyde or other neurotoxins that are within that vaccine. It may be receiving several vaccines at the same time. We were talking about the toxic load. It may be that you get five vaccines at once, your ability as a young child as an infant to handle all of those at once maybe compromised because you don't have glutathione, because you don't have the antioxidants because you're otherwise ill, with atopic autoimmune or gastrointestinal condition.

As we've talked about there are many chemicals, pesticides, etc. that are problematic for our susceptible children. But one thing that we are doing in our foods is genetically modifying them. Genetically modified foods are more able to handle pesticides, so a food that is a GMO food actually has more exposure to pesticides than other foods. So again without even knowing it we may be exposing our children to higher levels of those chemicals, which they are unable to handle.

Roundup is a chemical that many of us have been exposed to in our homes or in our environment that may be one of those other chemicals that disrupted the metabolism very early on either prenatally or immediately postnatally of our children, disturbing their methylation and sulfation to such a degree that then they were predisposed to more problems later.

DB: Can children recover from autism?

NHO: Children can recover from autism. It's not universal but if they have many triggers, many early problems and we can intervene early enough and help the gastrointestinal, the immunologic, and metabolic problems that they have; some of these children can recover.

✳ ✳ ✳

I know this was a lot of information for you to take in all at once. As you may have noticed, I purposely ask each of the practitioners some of the same questions, so the most vital facts are repeated from a different perspective, and the information will resonate more with you and sink in a little deeper.

Dr. Nancy O'Hara is extremely knowledgeable about prevention in the areas of preconception, pregnancy, and for babies postnatally, and I followed many of the specific guidelines that she outlines above during the three years that I cleaned out prior to getting pregnant with my daughter. You may not need to go through as lengthy a process as I did, but please remember that I already had a child on the spectrum at home. I did all the testing that she mentioned throughout this interview. I took out foods that I was allergic to including gluten and dairy, and supplemented with probiotics, vitamin D, and fish oil among other things. My diet consisted mostly of organic whole foods and I significantly limited the amount of processed food. I changed all my personal care products and household cleaners to ones that were more natural and holistic.

One of the most important gifts that I gave my daughter was a natural childbirth. To this day it is way up there on a short list of things that I am most proud that I have done for her. I tried to breastfeed for as long as I could and when that was not working any longer, I started making the homemade Weston A. Price baby formula recipe. Here is the link: **http://www.westonaprice.org/ childrens-health/formula-homemade-baby-formula/.**

You can see the nutritional information in the table chart and compare it to other baby formulas. I like that this recipe includes some very nutritious ingredients like coconut oil, olive oil, vitamin C, cod liver oil, and probiotics. I am still horrified that I fed my son a formula that had so many ingredients listed that I could not even pronounce or simply understand. Many of them were obviously chemicals. So making that formula is another beautiful gift that I gave her. My husband and I sat in the kitchen late at night every three days and made enough to last until the next batch. This is something we are both so intensely proud of.

There have been times that I have even suggested to friends that have children with constant ear infections or asthma to try taking milk out, since it can be a very common trigger. They have flat out told me "it's too hard." I think nothing is too inconvenient if it means improving the quality of your child's life. This is probably the reason that I was able to get my son talking again seven years after his fateful stroke. Prevention is one of the most important things you can do and nothing is more beautiful than to witness the extraordinary healing process as well.

CHAPTER SUMMARY:

Diet should be anti-inflammatory, consisting of organic protein, fruits, vegetables, nuts, and seeds.

Detoxify your environment by getting rid of chemicals in personal care products and household cleaners. Inspect your home for possible heavy metal contamination and consider testing yourself for it as well.

Have yourself checked for allergies or autoimmune, especially thyroiditis, which is very common in women who go on to have a child diagnosed with autism.

Make sure that you are having at least one bowel movement a day and, if not, speak to your practitioner about taking a natural supplement to help with this issue.

Consider having some simple testing done such as MTHFR, reduced glutathione, and homocysteine.

A natural childbirth is best but if it is not possible then make sure to take a probiotic or give probiotics to your baby if you're not able to breastfeed.

Speak to your practitioner about supplementing with probiotics, glutathione, essential fatty acids, and vitamin D.

Hyperbilirubinemia may be a red flag at birth without an ABO incompatibility with mom and without excessive dehydration.

A child with eczema, atopic dermatitis, food allergies, colic, yeast rash or thrush, reflux, chronic constipation, or recurring ear infections may be displaying an early sign that their immune system is compromised.

Keep stress at bay as best as you can.

Chapter 6

NUTRITION

PRECONCEPTION, PREGNANCY AND BABY
with Geri Brewster, RDN, MPH, CDN

I think people are really beginning to catch on to how important diet is to one's overall health and well-being. There is still an overwhelming majority of the public who hang on to the notion that one has nothing to do with the other. I was among that majority for many years—it's natural to assume a food is safe and healthy if it's neatly packaged on a supermarket shelf, with a stamp that says "FDA Approved" on it. The media have been perpetuating this false narrative that chemicals and preservatives in your food are perfectly fine. In reality, they are just echoing what their advertisers and sponsors want them to say; granted some of them may not even know better. But what most people don't understand is that food companies are extremely powerful and they pay the media handsomely in advertising dollars. We no longer live in times where you can expect the governmental agencies like the FDA or EPA to look out for your best interest either. You are going to have to be your own watchdog and do the research yourself. The good news is that we are going to get you started here in this book, and then give you resources to continue collecting the latest information on disease prevention and holistic health, so you can continue to protect yourself and your children.

It has taken me many years to cultivate sources that can be trusted for real and accurate information about true health. Like most people, I thought if it was in a peer-reviewed article, then it should be accepted as gospel. However, I now understand that even scientists can be encouraged to write articles that are favorable to an outcome a food company desires for a particular product of theirs. In some cases the company even funds the study themselves. A former president of the *Lancet*, one of the most prestigious medical journals, has come out publicly admitting that many of the studies that doctors read are not necessarily authentic, but ghostwritten and paid for by pharmaceutical companies with vested interests in the outcome of what the study recommends. This isn't to say that all studies cannot be trusted. It just means that we need to pay close attention to the origin of our information, if the author has any conflicts of interest, and whether or not a big corporation has paid for the study.

Another issue is that people are being told by their doctors that what they eat really doesn't matter that much and what they really need is a pill to lower their cholesterol or to take care of their high blood sugar. Meanwhile functional medicine practitioners have known for decades that you can heal yourself from a variety of ailments and prevent them just by making some important changes to your diet. A pill may help alleviate your unwelcome symptoms in the short term, however it will most often just be suppressing the symptom. This can create a bigger issue when the problem begins to fester and get worse over time, since you are not addressing what has created it in the first place. You may also even experience one or many adverse side effects from these drugs. And the worst part is that once you start taking some of these pills, you need to stay on them for a very long time, lest you experience your original symptoms—possibly even in a more advanced state.

I applaud you for picking up this book in hopes of learning what you can do to prevent an illness before it begins. You are one of a growing group of people in this latest movement that does not want to perpetuate the status quo and keep following the SAD (standard American diet), or put yourself at risk by surrounding yourself with toxins in your personal care products and household cleaners. And many of you are not interested in band-aid medicine, where you have to stay on pills for most of your life. You can make a difference in your health now and clean things up before you really have a problem, and prevent your child from experiencing the pain of a chronic illness—especially one as devastating as autism.

It doesn't matter how old you are and what you have done in the past. The body has an amazing ability to heal itself and it wants to stay in balance, so give it the things that it needs to nourish itself now and you will soon experience the positive effects for years to come. From time to time, I cringe when I think back to some of the things I used to eat or slather on myself. I ate a lot of processed food growing up in the '70s and '80s. My family had a microwave that we used often. I now fully comprehend how dangerous microwaves are and would never consider using one. However, just like everyone else, I used to store leftover Chinese food in plastic and heat it up right in that plastic dish. Microwaves leach harmful chemicals including melted plastic into your food, as well as denaturing your food. Don't defeat your own best intentions after investing time cooking a healthy meal with lots of organic vegetables and spices, only to put it in a microwave, which zaps all the nutrients right out of it. I am proud that neither one of my children have ever experienced microwaved food. We stopped using one right before Dylan was born. I love my toaster oven. It cooks and heats up food very quickly without the microwave radiation.

If you just start changing little things here and there, then it will become easier to change the bigger items over time. You will notice a difference and be more open to these other changes. It is like a domino reaction. But don't feel like you have to do it all at once. You don't want to overload yourself and burn out from the added stress. Take your time. Even one small change a week will add up over time, and pretty soon you will have a much healthier lifestyle for you and your family. But most importantly you will feel more alive and your children will be healthier.

Now we dive into nutrition, a topic for which I have chosen a very special, experienced practitioner. Geri Brewster is so passionate and enthusiastic about nutritional prevention and healing. She has compiled such a wealth of knowledge in her many years of experience, and continues to educate herself and seek out new information daily to help her clients. Geri treats some of the most difficult cases from children with G-tubes to adults suffering from advanced MS (multiple sclerosis) or fibromyalgia.

I owe a lot of gratitude to Geri for helping me with both of my children and advising me during my preconception clean-up process. She has always been a gentle support, especially during my second pregnancy and when Jessica had her setbacks. I feel very lucky to share her expertise with all of you.

Geri Brewster, RDN, MPH, CDN, is a registered dietitian-nutritionist who works with adults and children in her practice using an integrative and personalized approach. She began her clinical career specializing in children and young adults with developmental disabilities and complex feeding issues. She maintains advanced studies in the fields of nutrition, integrative medicine, and public health and speaks on these subjects often. Most recently, Geri has developed a new product line, Build Your Best Bump, which is aimed at helping couples promote a healthier pregnancy.

DB: Do you think the incidence of autism is increasing?

GB: Without a doubt autism is increasing.

DB: When did you first notice the change?

GB: I remember that as a consultant to many residential schools for multiply-handicapped children and group home environments, I began to notice a massive increase in the incidence of autism. As being part of the team and sitting down with the social workers, medical directors, OT (occupational therapist), PT (physical therapist), speech people and looking at referral packets, I remember we were all commenting on the changes in the referral packets. We went from a having maybe a single child with microcephaly, poor feeding skills, and who were nonverbal, to then what seemed to escalate to the point where we were getting packets of children daily who did not physically appear to have anything wrong with them, but were nonverbal, perseverative, obstinate in many ways, could not transition, had fits of rage, fecal smearing, self-injurious behavior, and attempting to consume inedible objects.

DB: You mentioned to me that the day-to-day job responsibilities of school nurses has been changing over the years. Could you tell us more about that?

GB: Years ago, your average school nurse was there to provide a band-aid or the occasional medication distribution; now they're essentially infirmaries, distributing meds to kids routinely (daily), and addressing learning issues, behavioral issues, allergy and medical issues. Sometimes, it involves doing all of the above.

DB: Do you see a lot more sick children in your practice than you did years ago?

GB: In terms of closely examining the increase in autism diagnosis, it really parallels the increase in chronic illness in children across the board. The children whom I am seeing now, unfortunately, I do feel are sicker—and assuming we're comfortable using the word recovery, I would say that I think it's harder to provide treatment/assistance to enable these children to recover. There were many children whom I began with twenty years ago that were nonverbal and stimming (self-stimulating), sick a lot, with regular occurrence of ear infections and early antibiotic exposure, etc., who have managed to make their way into college environments and really achieve phenomenal successes, especially considering how rocky the first five years of their lives were.

Again, I've noticed that it has become tougher over the years to implement those same recommendations and provide the support necessary to get the kind of response that was once achieved. It certainly seems to make sense that their parents were just a little bit more exposed and perhaps grew up without the healthiest cell division and hence may not have served as the ideal hosts for a child coming into the world. These parents may have come in through C-section or had early antibiotic exposure. Those contributors could add up creating that initial perfect storm for that little baby not to have their neurological and immune system get a strong foothold. This then leads to significant dysregulation of the immune system from an early onset.

DB: A lot of people talk about the idea that parents today are being exposed to more toxins than the generation before, and that this exposure has resulted in otherwise healthy women not being able to conceive naturally on their own without the assistance of IVF, hormone therapy, etc. Is there a connection?

GB: It's striking to me how much more compromised the parents' immune systems are (especially the mother's) going into the procreation process today than in decades past. I'm looking at a mom, who had her child at thirty-six, and who had been on medications, in one form or another from the time that she was sixteen. Also, she had a lot of soft signs of an overreactive immune system, like eczema and asthma, yet she was considered just fine—people with these types of early signs were considered very normal, and those women were likely never told by their OBGYN or general practitioner of these possible contributors.

For instance, young women today go off to college with their inhaler, steroid cream, birth control pill, Prilosec™, Zoloft™, and maybe Adderall™. This is everyday America. That's on top of whatever that girl was exposed to in the twenty years prior, and as we've been talking about one's exposure to all these contributors has been increasing with time. A lot of the food that you feel is healthy is preprepared somewhere else, so we don't know exactly what it's been exposed to. It could be loaded with sulfites or preservatives. It's not coming from your kitchen or your garden. Then you have a few antibiotics each year, a few yeast infections, which you treat with Diflucan™ or Monistat™. For years and years, the standard protocol is to treat the symptoms, but never the root causes. You can see how all these factors add up—and can cause all kinds of issues down the road for their children, and their children's children, and so on.

DB: What are some of the other factors that make it more difficult to conceive?

GB: We certainly know the endocrine disruptors from a lot of the chemical plasticizers and even pesticides that run interference with our endocrine system. It's all closely connected: the immune system, neurological system, and endocrine system. Those three systems are always cross-talking. We certainly know that there are many estrogen mimickers in these plastics and there's an estrogen dominance that can inhibit conception. It will reduce testosterone levels in males, lowering sperm counts. You need enough progesterone on board to attain and maintain a pregnancy, and that's really hard to come by when these estrogen mimickers are introduced into human bodies.

We also need a good fat base in our diet as a woman to hold a pregnancy. When you look at how adulterated the fats in our food supply have been, it's only recently that trans fats have been taken out of most products in our food supply. People are now aware of how dangerous they are and it's almost like they never existed. When they were taken out of the food supply, the focus was on the cardiovascular risks that became so well known. However, we fail to acknowledge that vascularization includes our brain and everything leading up to our brain.

Supplement companies began adding fat components to standard prenatal vitamins. They started with first adding DHA, which is an essential omega-3 fatty acid as recently as 2000, which was also added to formulas and baby foods. This occurred because everyone was afraid to consume eggs. In turn people weren't receiving healthy levels of DHA from their egg yolks. So DHA, choline and now serine are all being added. Phosphatidylserine is even available as a prescription medical food to help as a non-stimulant treatment for children with ADHD, impulsivity and poor regulation. These are nutrients that would have once been found in egg yolks and organ meats. Bone broths are also making a big come back because the idea is we're looking for these nourishing nutrients to get them back into our bodies for the sake of future generations.

DB: What are the most important things that you might speak with a pregnant client about?

GB: I would look at the prenatal vitamin and the quality of the nutrients in that prenatal vitamin, especially the folate source and form. Considering we now know that about forty percent of the population is not equipped genetically to methylate their folate, I think as a pregnant individual, you really want to look at having a methylfolate, not folic acid (which is synthetic), in that prenatal vitamin. You want to make sure she's getting DHA, either part of the prenatal vitamin or separately. Choline is very essential to early neurological development and that choline should be supplemented as well.

Along the lines of the growing difficulties in conception, even miscarriages are on the rise, and a healthy amount of methylatefolate is necessary in order to maintain a pregnancy. I tell a lot of women who've had a couple of miscarriages—they either need to get on a methylfolate or they should at least do the testing for the MTHFR mutations.

DB: What are some of the things that you recommend women do who want to get pregnant and how far in advance should they be following your advice?

GB: For at least three months preconception, I recommend a low inflammatory diet and that involves the removal of inflammatory foods like gluten, casein, and soy. I recommend avoiding all GMOs, and encouraging a low inflammatory, high antioxidant foods that have high Omega-3s. A woman considering conception should be careful with fish selection—I use the seafood watch list. We have to be careful about the wild fish, certainly for the mercury and contaminants, that we want to avoid. We also need to be careful with farmed fish, because of the hormones and antibiotics that are pumped into them at some of these fisheries, although now we are starting to see some organically farmed fish. If something carries the organic label and the verified non-GMO label, I would say it's probably a safe bet. Getting blood sugar under control and reducing excess carbohydrates in an effort to reduce insulin levels, because insulin is a pro-inflammatory hormone, are also really helpful in improving chances of a natural conception.

If we have the luxury of looking at lab test results, I recommend testing for baseline inflammatory markers like sedimentation rate and C-reactive protein. I think in three months, you can rebuild a good amount of your body, and you have to do it in that nice slow way because you don't want to do a major detox. Your body must be prepared to eliminate those toxins, so you don't want to flood the mom's bloodstream with them.

Again, I like to suggest at least three months prior to conception for a multitude of reasons, to do it slowly, methodically and let some of these changes really then get incorporated as one's lifestyle changes. You want to remove all the offending factors and you want to replete with all these good nutrients before conception. This is also, not only for the health of the baby, but then for the health of the mother post-baby. A woman's health will very often significantly decline in those first couple of years after the birth of a baby, because you're busy taking care of an infant, and also if you're nursing the body gets depleted of essential nutrients.

DB: What types of problems are you constantly seeing with kids today that weren't prevalent in years past? And how have things changed nutritionally over the years?

GB: Anxiety disorder. I remember sitting at this very table we're currently sitting at. A seven-year-old boy came in with his mom after I had seen the mom a couple of times, and we had been making some alterations to his diet. She said he was ready to meet me because he wanted to really talk to me about how he feels when he eats certain foods. He came in and he had a hard time even making eye contact. He said "I have . . ." and his mom was like, "Look up, look at her." He looked up and then he went back down. Then without looking up he said, "I know I should be making eye contact, but you know it's hard for me because I have a lot of anxiety."

Honestly, I felt my heart drop because at that moment, I remembered the first time that I became aware in my own body of anxiety. I was thirty-two years old when I realized at one point with my type-A, uber-efficient, outcome-oriented personality that some of that was being driven by anxiety and I identified that as part of a personality aspect rather than a disorder. But I was in my early thirties, it's fairly normal for someone at that age—confronted with the challenges and decisions I had to make at that time—to experience anxiety in that way. I thought it was tragic for a seven-year old, for his childhood to be hijacked by a mental health disorder, because he should be so liberated and feel so safe and secure at this age. But he didn't. He had sleep problems, attention problems, and he was medicated. I'm happy to say he's much older now and he's not medicated, but it's taken a lot of work.

He was also totally a white-bread-and-milk kid. It took a lot to talk him into being open to shifting his diet. It's not so much for him to have to know the science behind it at such a young age, but at least be willing to cooperate with some type of behavioral plan to go along with it in an effort to give his brain a little bit of a break. Sometimes it's as simple as looking at the food that's going in and the behavioral and physical output and recognizing we're not going to get a different output unless we just change the food that's going in.

Even if we haven't done a whole lot of testing, sometimes it's just worth changing things up and seeing what we get. In his case, I came to know, as his mom did, that the components of that "white" diet were more excitatory. It was a low-protein diet too. I'm sure low blood sugar had a lot to do with his anxiety.

DB: Do you think the way children learn can contribute to anxiety?

GB: I remember going to a back-to-school night when my youngest was in middle school and one of the teachers, of course, was using those smart boards for the parent presentation. There was one in front of us, one to the side, and he is jumping back and forth between screens. I'm thinking to myself, "Oh my gosh, this is how kids are learning." They're learning at such a faster pace, but that can drive your adrenaline. You're in that constant state of fight and flight, which inhibits melatonin production later in the day and interrupts sleep cycles. The amount of technology people interact with on a daily basis has skyrocketed in this last decade like never before. We still don't know what the fallout is going to be from this exposure. But I can tell you there has absolutely been an increase in anxiety disorder across the board for almost every kid that I see.

DB: Besides technology changing, you talk about how some of our simple foods that have always been around have changed. Please explain the example that a piece of pizza is no longer like a piece of pizza I had growing up?

GB: I talk about pizza, as it comes up very often and just about everyone can relate. In fact, just this past week I saw a family whose mom reported how well her child had been doing after two weeks on a gluten-free casein-free diet, from a behavioral standpoint. Then one weekend she decided that one slice of pizza would be a nice treat. She thought, "We used to live on this, how much could it really hurt?" The fallout from that single slice was multiple tantrums, difficulty transitioning, and a huge increase in aggression.

What I reminded her is that sure, there's the casein and gluten that could be both inflammatory and or excitatory. A local pizzeria thirty years ago might have still been making their own dough. Most of them now are purchasing it. It's has dough conditioners and preservatives in there to maintain it. Years ago, there were some Italian family member in the back shredding the fresh mozzarella. Now it comes pre-shredded with mold inhibitors and other chemical agents out of a plastic bag. It's the chemical load on top of the gluten and the casein that's being introduced into a child's digestive system or bloodstream. The more processed food becomes and the older it is from its original starting point, the more free glutamate is in that food, the more histamines are in that food, which get metabolized as excitatory neurotransmitters on their way out of the body. You experience a huge excitatory inflammatory assault from eating a highly processed food.

The subsets of people that used to react to foods suddenly have exploded. Maybe because our guts are a little leakier, we're getting more of a flood into our bloodstream and then our blood brain barriers are a little more permeable as well. A leaky gut is more permeable because it may not have had the best footprint from a bacterial standpoint right out of the gate, so it never really got a good foothold. So, some of these whole proteins can enter the bloodstream more easily, which sets up an inflammatory response in the body. And then there is a leaky blood brain barrier. Some of these chemical compounds are taken up into the brain. We know that these compounds can influence the brain and there are subsets of people who may have been vulnerable to these chemicals if they ate certain foods.

DB: Tell me about how food has changed. What's been introduced in the last fifteen years that's so different than when I grew up that might be affecting children today?

GB: Besides just the structural changes that occurred with hydrogenating fats, we've seen a lot more sugar added which really serves as a preservative in many ways. This is why baked goods or a cookie can last on the shelf. They have a two-year shelf life and a cookie is kind of indestructible. Think about that. How could we expect to break it down and assimilate it in our body if it's basically indestructible and can't spoil.

Food companies have been molecularly altering our food by taking corn and converting it into a syrup. Then taking a fat and hydrogenating it to make it like a lard so that these foods could hang out forever without getting rancid or a stale taste. We've also genetically modified many of these core crops, soy and corn in particular, which wind up in a majority of processed foods. The wheat products, while they're not specifically genetically modified, have been hybridized and they've been made virtually indestructible by the addition of glyphosate so that they're so resistant to break down from all the pests and fungi. You can put wheat in a silo and it could be there for two years, it comes out and then it gets all refined. When you eat something that is flour-based, it could be a couple of years old already.

DB: What is it that agricultural companies promised us would occur with making GMOs? And then tell us what you have seen occur.

GB: It was all under the banner of feeding the hungry, and the promise of how genetically modified fish can feed all the starving people in the world today. I think there are other ways that we could figure out to feed all the starving people in the world without genetically restructuring our food in a way that may be unrecognizable to the body, and hence set up more inflammation or potentially change the transcription and replication within the bacteria in the gut in response to being exposed to that food. That gut bacteria are going to proliferate and modulate our immune, neurological, and endocrine systems.

After World War II when we added antibiotics and steroids to the food supply, it was one thing to add them for medical purposes— undeniably they saved a lot of lives. It all started getting dumped in the food supply. Of course, it then changed the guts of all the animals. And we started ingesting all the genetically modified food from feeding that to all the animals, which wouldn't have been their natural diet. A cow doesn't walk up to a stalk of corn and start gnawing on it. This changed their guts. It made them sicker, and then of course it changes their stool. So, they're getting an overgrowth of bad bacteria in their guts, and they are stepping in their own unhealthy manure and some of that gets cross-contaminated in the slaughterhouses with the food supply.

I do think unfortunately that profitability triumphs over everything, and I just think we should come up with some form of real ethical capitalism and that profitability should be tied hand-in-hand with the health and well-being of the people and the planet. That's the only way we're going to survive as a species and as a planet.

DB: You have performed a lot of assessments of patients, health histories who come in with autism. What are the commonalities among many of these children? We refer to them as contributors and then many times there's a trigger, that straw that broke the camel's back. I look back at Dylan and I could come up with like thirty contributors and I could think of a couple triggers. What are these common contributors that you have seen looking over a child's health history?

GB: The common contributors I would have to say include inflammation in a mom, generally high sugar, high stress, and maybe poor sleeping—which of course is a by-product of high stress and sugar. Within the baby, I think birth process, C-section very often too, it's not all cases, but very often I think that when a mother requires some type of reproductive endocrinologist facilitation for that pregnancy, it can often be a contributor. The goal is accomplished and it's a wonderful thing then to have that pregnancy outcome. I know from some of the moms that have come to me while maybe approaching their third failed IVF that their percentage of body fat and the quality of their diet were questions that were not even asked before they went into that hormonal protocol.

I have definitely helped to optimize a woman's health and whether that was the reason that their next IVF was successful I don't know, but I'd like to think it helped. You have to always optimize nutritional status. A woman loses her period when the body is threatened, underweight, or experiencing too much stress. That period stops, because the body knows you can't support a pregnancy and you need a minimum of fourteen percent body fat to maintain a period and that's because the body has to have enough fat to then deliver to that early neurological system.

It's almost like the universe is telling us all now that you're having all these procreation problems because we're not supposed to be procreating because we're just not in a good place to do so. We pushed our way through, with the miracles of modern science, then sometimes it shows up in the pregnancy outcome.

DB: Tell me what patients say they feel are the triggers. For Dylan, a trigger that only I would know was he was eating an enormous amount of gluten in the two months prior. His addiction just stepped up ten-fold. We gave it to him more freely but he was asking for it all the time, and it seemed to calm him down at first. I did not understand the concept at the time that people can crave foods that they are allergic to.

GB: He was probably one of the kids who had more of an opioid response.

DB: It was like heroin to him. Then the second trigger was that he had a Hib vaccine at eighteen months, which caused an ischemic stroke. He had two major triggers, but it was also the thirty things that led up to that. Dylan was diagnosed with failure to thrive. He also experienced many of the soft signs such as red cheeks, spit up, undiagnosed food allergies, you name it. He had everything including eczema, drooling, the rash around the penis, and yeast. What are the triggers that you notice and that parents talk about?

GB: Well, certainly everything that you just described for Dylan, unfortunately that's not an uncommon scenario. And a lot of parents do feel it was an illness or a vaccine that was just the final straw. I know the discussion on vaccine is so hotly debated and it's hard to even bring it up or to go there without invoking any kind of emotional or political or legal reaction. It's just the idea that it's there to shift the immune system to respond. Knowing the level of complications that could occur when we're faced with any type of pathogen, whether it's a natural exposure or a vaccine, an accidental exposure or a purposeful exposure, that it's going to trigger an immune response. If our immune system is strong enough and capable, it'll do the right thing. If it's not, it's going to succumb either to that illness or possibly it'll turn into another illness.

When someone is vaccinated, you are bypassing the priming of the immune system. It's like coming in the back door. This doesn't only relate to children, either. We've had the discussion regarding Gulf War soldiers. If your body is really not prepared or supported and you then overload it and expect that immune system to respond properly, it can succumb. As far as Gulf War syndrome, was it related to chemical exposures in the field or the vaccinations, or all of it? A total load? The idea is that the immune system imploded.

Much of what we're vaccinated against are diseases that you would breathe in, droplet and airborne, so that would give all of your first line of defense an opportunity to try to fight it. Your cilia, mucus membranes, and your secretory IgA (immunoglobulin A), or at least that you're sending those chemical signals to the rest of the immune system that something might be coming, so you're priming it.

When you're taking it in a vaccine, you're not being primed, it's coming in the back door. You're slammed right away. It's possible that it could set up a hyperreactive response to that germ and the rest of the body. I also know in discussions with many immunologists, they can't really answer that question either, because the immune system seems to really be shifting in response to all these epigenetic and environmental factors because the heavy metals, pollutants, and pesticides in our environment have really changed our immune system. We didn't always react to as much as we do today. The allergy numbers are just as high in diagnosis as autism, so there's clearly a hyper response in our immune system these days. Why is that happening? Nobody can answer that. As long as nobody can answer that, I don't really see how anybody definitively could say that any kind of illness, sickness, or vaccine doesn't necessarily contribute to the total load of a child developing another disease.

What we do know now from the whole genomics understanding of the human genome that again from our immune response, some of us are going to be genetically predisposed to having an adverse reaction because we just cannot manage being exposed to something directly into our bloodstream that way.

DB: What have parents said to you in regard to vaccines?

GB: The reason I even went into the whole discussion with regards to the vaccines is because there are many parents who do feel that was the ultimate trigger. They are constantly hearing from physicians, the media, publications that there's absolutely no connection. They're so baffled and some feel very betrayed by that. Because they know their child and they talk about the regression, losing their child and seeing that happen in the weeks and months following specific vaccines. From all my reading, the best that I could do is tell them exactly what I told you, so at the very least, they're not feeling like they're crazy. I also want them to have an appreciation of all these biochemical nuances.

DB: Do you think autism can be prevented?

GB: I absolutely think autism can be prevented because I do think that autism in some instances is a result of a total load where there's just total inflammation going on and the brain is inflamed. I can't speak to this as well as a neurologist may be able to. But certainly, something is running interference with the normal pruning process of a young infant brain because the brains of children with autism have been found to be larger. That largeness is really a lack of pruning and synaptic connectivity from this generalized inflammation to me.

I also know from many of the families that I worked with where parents were quite certain that a younger sibling was fast tracking into an autism diagnosis. Had we not begun the work on the sibling, using those same recovery strategies for the older sibling who was diagnosed, parents really felt that it was completely responsible for then preventing the ultimate diagnosis.

DB: A lot of mothers like myself were sick at the time when they had their baby and didn't think it had any bearing on the child. I had multiple chemical sensitivities at the time, which I now know was from leaky gut, mercury toxicity, and a vaccine reaction to a tetanus shot. Next I force myself to get pregnant with Dylan through IVF. I'm the classic story. Can we talk a little bit about mom's being sick and how that affects the baby?

GB: There is a lot that goes on in terms of immune sharing. Sometimes I take a family history and mom has got significantly noted food allergies for which she avoided those known food allergies during pregnancy. However, it doesn't mean that she didn't have a leaky gut, other food sensitivities, and inflammation going on that were never addressed. Here her little one is now being born and sensitive to everything, reactive to everything and diagnosed ultimately with eosinophilic esophagitis, failure to thrive and ultimately needing an elemental formula.

Suddenly we have all these children with eosinophilic esophagitis (EOE). People are asking, "Did it always exist?" I have parents who are actually being told that because the EOE is being kept under control by the child being on Nexium™, Prevacid™, or Prilosec™, that it's fine for them to even eat the foods that are associated with EOE from an allergy standpoint. "Because we're suppressing the symptoms, it's okay to give the food," is the general mind-set. I don't condone that stance, because that food is probably not going to help, another area of the body may then get inflamed, and just because we're keeping the inflammation down in the esophagus with suppression (with a proton pump inhibitor which is also running interference now with that child's ability to absorb B vitamins and minerals for the rest of its life) it doesn't mean we're solving the problem.

We're not looking at the whole nutritional picture of this child for a lifetime. Here was a mom with a history of food allergies who didn't eat those allergenic foods during pregnancy but still had a child who was born with severe food allergies. She's just thinking it's all related to genetics. There's genetic predisposition, but you can see how the inflammatory cascade may have induced this kind of manifestation in her child.

DB: How has the microbiome changed in recent years?

GB: We've altered it dramatically because we've altered our food supply so dramatically. We can appreciate the benefits of probiotics and the importance of supplementing with them. It's because we don't have what we need due to a lack in our diets of fermented foods. And we're also being exposed to antibiotics and steroids directly and indirectly through our food.

We've altered farming practices and the usage of pesticides in conventional farming practices have increased in use changing the soil microbes that impact our immune system. This relates to the hygiene theory, in which we're killing all of our microbes—good and bad—with the antimicrobial soaps, alcohol-based hand-sanitizers, etc. When you talk about the farming communities and children that were raised on farms and with farm animals, they could have been touching animal manure and not necessarily washing their hands but never getting sick as a result of that exposure. There was a symbiosis that was working, and if anything, some of those germs so to speak helped their immune system respond appropriately.

DB: Why is it so important to expose children to the right germs early on?

GB: When children are crawling around on the floor, parents say, "Well, they're supposed to get a certain amount of dirt." I think, "They're supposed to be getting clean dirt (pardon the oxymoron), not crawling around the floor in Macy's where the concern is more toxins that they're being exposed to as opposed to innocuous soil microbes. It's similar to what I hear some parents say about day care, in that it's supposed to be good for them; it exposes them to germs so that their immune system builds up. The idea that exposure to a lot of germs, like in the day care environment, that it's supposed to make a child a little hardier and more resilient, would be great if in fact it does, but unfortunately, many of them are constantly on antibiotics. If you're relying on antibiotics, which can be life-saving and necessary at times, you're not making your own immune system hardier and more resilient. We're not really gaining what we were hoping to achieve. The idea or the message is well-intentioned, but in reality, it's not what's happening.

DB: There is a lot of confusing information out there for parents regarding food allergies and what to feed their baby. I remember being given information with Dylan that conflicted with everything I did for my daughter. Could you break it down and explain from a nutritionist's standpoint how you like to see foods introduced?

GB: This is something that I discuss with parents a lot because over the years the American Academy of Pediatrics has changed its recommendations with regard to first foods. Right now, there is still a little bit more of a movement toward early introduction, almost as a means of desensitization. But if a child's reactive, then unfortunately again once that reactivity is ignited it's really hard to settle that kind of reactivity to food.

So, thirty-five years ago, you were told to not introduce any of the known allergens until one year of age and older, and now we're starting to see some allergens are being introduced early as I said from a desensitization standpoint. Solids and high allergens are two different things. Solids were introduced as early as three months. It might still even be as early as three months, somewhere in that three- to six-month range for first introduction of foods. I think generally we're always trying to encourage families not to begin until six months of age.

When it comes to more allergenic foods like milk, it's still not recommended until one year, as again it's a large molecular protein.

And that has shifted in the more recent years to maybe earlier intro-duction, because all these allergies were developing, so the thought was if there was early introduction it would be a way for there to be some desensitization similar to now what's proposed with regard to peanut allergy. To prevent anaphylaxis if there is concern or family history, then through an early type of skin testing, if reaction occurs to then use some transdermal exposure from several months of life for the body to become friends essentially with the protein, so that if there is exposure later it's not such a shock to the immune system that it goes into an anaphylactic reaction.

I know that there are recommendations for some early introduc-tions now, but if there is a history in the family of food allergy, those allergens are still recommended to wait until later. Egg white protein is a high allergen so I think it's often best to still wait until after one year of age, rather than run the risk of a provocation early on, because as I've said from that cellular memory standpoint—once that allergy is in place, it has to be avoided for a very long period of time, and then very slow introduction thereafter for the body to be okay with it. It's some-thing that's very personalized, so the American Academy of Pediatrics and Pediatricians only have some general guidelines to follow.

I work collaboratively with pediatricians on the best feeding regi-men for that infant. Food has become very sophisticated and there are a lot of food combinations that are out there, say in stage one (first solid foods). This stage one may include puree organic strawberries and banana, but technically berries are a high allergen food. A mom could start giving it because it says stage one and then suddenly the child is flaring. You don't know whether the flare is an actual allergy response from the berry or is it from a salicylate or phenolic compound. Is it a flushing reaction? That's what also makes things confusing.

DB: What types of problems have you seen with this type of early introduction?

GB: I've had some parents come in and their kids are covered with eczema and they're maybe just a little over one and they've done a little bit of skin testing because the blood allergies don't show up that early in age. When I hear this in the food history, it's been a lot of sophisticated food very early on. They're coming to me to find out what we can feed our children. So, I just think it has to be very individualized and I do still take a very prudent approach toward food, early food introduction. I feel like the longer that you wait and get that good gut functioning and have a good solid immune and neurological integration and regulation going on, then we can deal with the stimulation of food from that chemical basis.

Personally, I do not like to see the grains introduced so early because we do know that grains in and of themselves can be very high inflammatory foods. They certainly cross react with all the grass allergies and so many kids have environmental spring allergies to trees and grasses. We often start with grains like rice cereal for iron fortification, because somewhere between three and six months of age, the baby's stored iron that it received from its mother begins to go down. They need more iron-rich sources. Unless you wanted to do a little bit of bone broth, you're going to traditionally go to these iron fortified cereals. But we don't have to, there are other iron-rich foods that can serve as first foods. And then at that point you can start supplementing with a good clean liquid multivitamin and iron source. It doesn't have to be in a cereal or a carbohydrate form.

I really prefer to introduce and recommend introducing vegetables first and then move into some of the fruits and the cooked meats, and then following up with the starchy root vegetables, like sweet potatoes. Then wait till you're getting closer to that one-year mark before introducing some of the gluten-free grains and just allow the integrity of the gut and all that and tolerance to these other foods to develop.

DB: What supplements do you think a mom needs to continue after the pregnancy?

GB: I've talked to a number of moms who didn't realize that they needed to take their prenatal vitamins while they were nursing. We need to make sure that we've got a nice enriched breast milk that's coming from nutrient dense foods but supplemental nutrients as well.

DB: What is bio-individuality and how does it translate into medicine?

GB: This microbiome within us is extremely significant and as we learn about it in combination with our own genomic mapping we can then ultimately personalize the best diet and introduce pharmaceuticals only when safe and necessary. That will become the personalized medicine of the future if we're going to survive as a species. You could have two patients of exactly the same demographics, sex, age, lifestyle, area, the same disease diagnosis, give them the same treatment protocol and one does well with it and one doesn't. What are the factors that exist that make up those differences that has everything to do with their individualized genomics and their individualized microbiome, which is going to then dictate how their immune system and all body systems respond to that drug?

DB: Many parents find their doctors are very resistant to an individualized protocol especially when it entails going on a "special diet" or allergy-free diet. Why do you think pediatricians have such trouble with parents trying a special diet?

GB: I think a number of reasons. One, special diets were always considered a fad so that gets minimized right away. I think that it's often thought we're running the risk of eliminating key nutrients. Unfortunately, when a child is only eating like five white foods, they're getting far fewer nutrients than when we switch over to say a more healing diet that might consciously eliminate some of those inflammatory foods, but are big on building up very nourishing foods. I also think maybe not everybody can have an appreciation of the science behind, it. I think all these factors impact why it's dismissed.

DB: Let's talk about the obesity epidemic, how it relates to the microbiome, and how it's a problem for children in this country today.

GB: We have this obesity epidemic going on with all the children in this country and several years ago the World Health Organization said this generation of children will be the first not to live as long as their parents. We've been increasing in longevity over the last couple of hundred years, but now it's believed we're going to take a backslide.

   This is not necessarily because they were speaking to the numbers of autism, allergies, and pediatric cancers as much as they were looking at chronic disease from an obesity, hypertension, heart disease standpoint. For so long we always heard calories in equal calories out, and the calorie is a calorie but it's not true at all.

   First, we metabolize different macronutrients, proteins, fats, and carbohydrates that are delivering calories at different rates. The rate at which our metabolism functions is dictated by our gut flora. You could have a child who's obese and they might be a couch potato. Or maybe they're just eating crappy food, but it still might only be 1,500 calories a day, and they might need to be getting two thousand. Yet they're blowing up because the crappy food that they're eating is serving as a substrate for some of the non-beneficial, the non-favorable metabolic–oriented bacteria in the gut. We're feeding the wrong bacteria. It's slowing down the metabolism and you're gaining weight even if you're not eating that much.

DB: Do you think that good nutrition can fix most children's chronic health issues?

GB: I believe in the healing power of food and I believe in the healing power of the body. When you are putting those healing foods or just good foods into the body, you have the power to turn around all kinds of disease.

I went into the field of nutrition because I believed in its healing power, but I went through a very conventional training in nutrition. What I was taught through very conventional training was that every disease had a special diet for it. Back in those days, you had diabetes, you had your diabetic diet. You had hypertension, you had your hypertensive diet.

I get referrals from physicians whom I never met because they are pleased with the outcomes and progress of patients that I've treated. Doctors do want to see their patients get better, they may not have the tools in their toolkit to help that patient because what the missing piece, despite all the medication, was really the nutritional care piece. I've been able to implement dietary changes and have great positive medical outcomes.

DB: Is prevention easier than trying to recover a child from autism?

GB: An ounce of prevention is worth a pound of cure. I think it's definitely always easier to prevent than to work toward recovery. That's why we want to stack the deck in a family's favor right from the get-go and that's why I think the preconception wellness and detoxification and inflammation reduction is so vital.

DB: Tell me a little bit about your supplement line?

GB: It's really an educational program for parents' preconception. The idea is that we just want to optimize our own health and then ultimately the health of future generations. Given the statistics, we seem to be losing in that area right now. Until we figure out another way, I've got to do everything I can to help couples to clean up their act; and they may not have even realized how much cleaning up their act was needed because very often we think we're doing the right thing but we may be exposing ourselves to quite a lot of environmental toxins. And we can all use a good low inflammatory diet and detoxification program for general health and well-being.

   We get that one chance to build your best bump. We can't make any pregnancy guarantees, but we want to make sure that we do the best we can to build that best bump because it's really hard after that delivery to go back as I said, the impact on a cellular level seems to be going deeper with every generation. I'm hoping this is an opportunity to turn that around so I don't have to have another mom or dad say to me, "We wish we had known."

As you see, nutrition plays such an important role in preventing chronic illness, especially one as overwhelming as autism. My advice would be to start making small changes such as limiting processed food and trying to buy as much organic as possible. There is nothing more important than giving your body the nutrition it deserves. Remember you will be passing along this solid nutrition in the way of your microbiome and immune system as it interplays with your baby in the womb. One of the greatest gifts that you can give your child is the tools to build a healthy immune system. They will have this gift for the rest of their life and pass it on to their own offspring.

CHAPTER SUMMARY:

Limiting processed foods is a great first step.

An anti-inflammatory diet is your best bet in preventing disease. Eat lots of fresh fruit, vegetables, protein, and seeds or nuts.

Buy organic as often as possible.

Avoid GMO food as much as possible. We have no idea how this will affect our DNA going forward for future generations.

Take care of your microbiome by eating fermented foods and/or supplementing with probiotics.

Remember symptoms are clues to what may be going on in your body—and symptoms should be examined holistically.

Using medicine in the short term can alleviate symptoms, but it won't get to the root of the problem.

Moms should stay on a multivitamin, mineral, or prenatal while they are nursing, not just for the baby but to give themselves the nutrients they need as well.

Be careful when introducing solid food to a baby. If your baby has shown signs of difficulty with formulas and breast milk, such as reflux, constipation, eczema, and rashes, then consider waiting on introducing high allergen foods. Discuss a customized plan with your pediatrician or dietitian-nutritionist.

The body has an incredible ability to heal, so give it the necessary tools to complete this task.

CHAPTER 7

KEEPING BABY SAFE
with Maureen McDonnell, RN

It takes a pretty large assault—or at least a multitude of smaller ones—to send a child cascading into the abyss of autism. Unfortunately, there are countless things that can come together to create this perfect storm, and some of them will be quite obvious, like not being outside if someone is directly spraying pesticides on a lawn, whereas others are less apparent. The purpose of this chapter is to get you thinking about the ones that might not be so obvious to you, but can still do enough damage nonetheless.

Nutrition is a wonderful and necessary start, however, there are many other things involved in creating an imbalance in the body that ultimately lead to an illness. Later in the book, we will discuss genetic variations that can put you at risk. Then one of the practitioners will explain the concept of epigenetics, when a gene that puts you at risk for cancer or an autoimmune gets turned on. Environmental toxins are a concept we have already touched on a little bit and will continue to investigate further. Now this brings us to some of the smaller things one does each day that can really add up and affect the outcome of your baby, whether or not they develop autism or some other childhood chronic illness.

I chose to speak with Maureen McDonnell, who has the unique perspective of having been a labor and delivery nurse, a certified childbirth educator, and has worked extensively in pediatrics as a holistic and nutritionally oriented RN for forty years. Maureen has truly seen it all. In 1998, she became the national coordinator for what was formerly known as the Defeat Autism Now! conferences. Theses seminars were instrumental in teaching parents and practitioners that autism is treatable and that recovery is possible. Currently, Maureen devotes most of her time as a health editor of a women's magazine, writing for various health publications and educating people about nutrition and the effects of the environment through an organization she cofounded: Saving Our

Kids Healing Our Planet (www.SOKHOP.com). I am extremely grateful she was able to take the time to speak with me.

DB: I always say that before we can talk about fixing or preventing a problem we need to recognize if there is one. I would like to ask if you think autism is increasing?

MM: I don't even know how emphatically I can express this. With all my heart and all my knowledge and all these years in pediatric nursing, without a doubt—a single doubt—the numbers have exploded. The autism rates have increased beyond belief. This idea that autism has always been around, that we just didn't know how to recognize it, is a fallacy. It's flat out not true.

When I was in nursing school in the late 1970s at Seton Hall University, near Newark, New Jersey, they had to bus nursing students for an hour to observe one child with autism. Now I could walk down the street here in Asheville, North Carolina, and meet five people, and at least one of them would know, or have, a child with autism. It's ludicrous to think that we had the same incidence or rates affecting children thirty years ago that we have today.

I also find it insulting to physicians, teachers, and nurses that were working with children thirty years ago to insinuate that they were somehow missing children with autism. They just weren't around. But today we really have an epidemic on our hands and it's time to look deeply at the reasons this is happening.

DB: Do you think autism can be prevented or at least minimize the risks?

MM: Yes. We love to blame disorders on genetics. But there's no such thing as a genetic epidemic. You can't have this many children affected by these problems and blame it on genes. I propose there may be some genetic component combined with an assault of environmental toxins, poor nutrition, and a huge increase in the number of vaccines causing this problem. There are a multitude of experienced experts in diverse areas of scientific disciplines that agree with me on this.

DB: You are a big proponent of the preconception clean out. How far in advance would you prefer that women get started with that process?

MM: When we speak about an ideal situation, I would say about a year prior to conceiving is best. The reason women need to do this is that the average woman is exposed to about five hundred potentially toxic ingredients in a day. For example, there can be over two hundred different chemicals in a single perfume. When you add that to the list of chemicals you find in deodorant, toothpaste, mascara, lipstick, shampoo, creams and lotions, fabric softeners, detergents etc., it's no wonder that so many women have a build up of toxins in their systems. Switching to more natural products is a great step in the right direction for a woman considering pregnancy.

Of course there are some toxins we can't avoid. However, the stronger a woman is nutritionally, the stronger her detoxification pathways are and the healthier her eliminative organs are, the better chance she has of avoiding a toxic build up thereby minimizing her and her babies health risks.

A child's entire immune system begins with its exposure to the mom's bacteria as he or she is passing through the birth canal. Supplementing with probiotics prior to conceiving and during pregnancy is another way the mom can positively impact the future health of her baby.

I have a strong belief that by addressing the underlying causes of health problems including depression and anxiety, and treating them with natural methods prior to conceiving, gives children the best chance of being unencumbered by the health problems that have become so common today.

DB: You mentioned in your article about how they're finding over one hundred different chemicals in cord blood of children today, can you speak a bit more about the importance of cleaning those chemicals out.

MM: That's right. We used to think that the placenta was just this perfect filter and protective barrier that it would not allow anything to get into the fetal blood system and into the body of the fetus. But the assault of chemicals is so much greater today that we can no longer solely depend on the placenta to filter the barrage of toxins that moms are currently exposed to.

DB: Why are these toxins in such a great number?

MM: In the past one hundred years we have created over 87,000 new chemicals and we have a chemical industry that has a very strong lobbying power in Washington, DC, so very few come off the market. Most of these chemicals have never been tested for their neurological, developmental, or behavioral impact on children. A newborn baby does not have the ability to detoxify these chemicals properly and their single and/or combined impact can have dire consequences.

DB: Let's talk about some of the smaller choices that occur during pregnancy and birth that can interrupt the natural birth process.

MM: Sure, like excessive ultrasounds during pregnancy, giving high doses of Pitocin during labor, separating the mom and baby after birth without allowing time for bonding and breastfeeding.

DB: Can we talk a little bit about Pitocin? It's used on so many women who enter hospitals. What's the issue when it comes to autism? How does it possibly increase the risk?

MM: Well, researchers don't have a clear understanding yet, but there does seem to be some problems with the oxytocin level of children with autism. Pitocin is a synthetic version of oxytocin, given to women in labor. It is a hormone that makes the contractions stronger and brings them on faster. Although sometimes necessary, it does interfere with the natural birth experience. Midwives are trained to be patient and have techniques that help a woman labor more effectively if things slow down. Those techniques are almost a lost art. In the natural childbirth classes I taught, using the Bradley method, it really wasn't encouraged to use anything artificial unless it was in an absolute dire emergency.

I chose to use midwives for my own two children, and all of my grandchildren's births were assisted by midwives. I'm not saying there's never an instance where Pitocin is necessary, but I think as with most medical procedures in labor and delivery, they can be used more for convenience rather than being patient and trusting the natural birth process.

DB: You've spoken in the past about the importance of writing down your birth plan. A lot of women have specific things in mind about how they want to give birth, and unfortunately they get to the hospital and some of them might be pressured to do things they didn't want to. Or the birth plan sometimes is altogether ignored. What can mothers do to help ensure their birth plan is carried out?

MM: Well that's such an important piece of the birth process. It starts with the mom doing her own research, reading, sharing, talking, and expressing her fears, concerns, and preferences.

I then suggest the couple sit down with the OBGYN or the midwife and go over their requests point by point. I used to have my childbirth students type out their list and have their birth attendant sign it. For many births, these preferences can and should be honored.

Moms are usually not the most communicative during labor, so it's a good idea for them to have either the dad, doula, or a friend be their advocate. If you're in a practice where there are multiple practitioners, then you have to make sure it's in your record and have it reviewed prior to going into labor, ensuring it's been signed off on. Some people might be concerned about what the labor nurse is going to think about them if they come in with a *list of preferences*? However those who are well-trained in the birthing field know that if God forbid there's an emergency, mom's preferences are no longer a top priority.

DB: Let's go back to the idea of preconception, since I think a lot of women don't understand that their health status prior to getting pregnant sometimes can keep them from getting pregnant or even cause a miscarriage. Geri Brewster touched on this a little bit.

MM: Women today are exposed to all these hormone-disrupting chemicals that exist, like parabens, phthalates, and formaldehyde. BPA (Bisphenol A) is another, which is a plasticizer in our plastic water bottles and is one particularly noteworthy chemical. The things we put on our body in the form of lotions contain a lot of chemical ingredients that disturb our hormones as well.

DB: Can you explain a little bit about how plastic and other endocrine disrupters can throw off our hormones?

MM: Certain chemicals mimic our own hormones. What that means is, there is a lock and key system on our cell membranes. If a hormone is attempting to get into the cell, but a chemical that looks like that hormone got there first and blocked the hormone's passage into the cell, well you can imagine the havoc that scenario causes.

We're now realizing that precocious puberty, infertility, polycystic ovary disease, and increased rates of breast cancer in women are due to the hormone disrupting components of the toxins in our environment, personal care products, cleaning products, and in our furniture or cars.

Besides certain chemicals causing hormonal imbalance, stress can also lead to dysregulation of our hormones. Stress, as we know, results in the production of cortisol, and when excess cortisol is being produced, the levels of other important hormones such as progesterone, DHEA, estrogen, etc., are reduced.

Approximately, ten to eleven percent of couples today experience problems with infertility and many have problems maintaining pregnancies. Some of these issues may also be related to a specific type of hormone imbalance referred to as "estrogen dominance" (caused by chemicals that mimic estrogen), which in turn causes a decrease in progesterone. Progesterone (pro-gest) is needed in order to maintain a pregnancy. Unfortunately, many couples are not aware of this issue.

DB: Let's talk about what some of the other maternal risk factors are that contribute and raise the risks of having a child with autism or chronic illness.

MM: We have the tried and true risk factors associated with poor health outcomes such as smoking, consuming alcohol, and taking illegal as well as some prescription drugs (such as antidepressants). And now we have access to more studies showing that antidepressant usage by pregnant mothers is really problematic in raising the risk of having a child with autism. I like to let moms know there are so many natural ways to improve depression, such as taking higher doses of omega-3, fatty acids, improving diet, balancing blood sugar levels, and giving the body the precursor nutrients it needs to manufacture serotonin (the neurotransmitter needed to battle depression). Also, gut health is of paramount importance, as eighty percent of serotonin production is in the gut. If you don't have a healthy gut, you're not going to be producing the right amount of serotonin, the neurotransmitter that keeps you in a good mood, helps you get a good night's sleep, and protects you from getting depressed.

Again, exposure to environmental toxins is a big risk factor because we know kids with autism are poor detoxifiers and their systems are overloaded. The Environmental Working Group has done studies that have found babies are now being born pre-polluted. Whether that turns into a problem where they have eczema, an auto-immune illness, autism, allergy, or asthma, it can't be good that these kids are being born with all of these chemicals in their system. We have to do all we can as mothers to make sure our risk factors are minimized prior to conception and birth. This can occur by eating organic food, not consuming anything that's genetically engineered, which has been sprayed with Roundup, which contains glyphosate. It's a horrible chemical that's destroying our gut flora. Drinking lots of filtered water not from a BPA plastic bottle, exercising, and getting our vitamin D all can help. Poor nutrition and environmental toxins are huge risk factors for excessive stress for pregnancy. I was reading this article the other day where the OBGYNs were essentially saying, "We emphasize a good diet and taking your prenatal vitamins, but we just can't get into the whole environmental thing because it's too overwhelming for our patients." To me, when something is this important, we as a society and our physicians better make time to educate our patients about all the risk factors.

DB: Let's talk a little bit more about why gut health is so important, especially for mothers who don't already have a child on the spectrum.

MM: The immune system is headquartered in the gut. If you have an issue, such as autism, anxiety, depression, or attention problems that involve the brain function, you've got to look at the gut because the neuro-transmitters are formulated there. So many of our health problems today start with the gut. As doctors Nancy O'Hara and Sid Baker, and many of us who were involved in the Autism Research Institute use the saying, "Heal the gut, Heal the child" as our mantra.

DB: What are some contributors to gut issues that you've taken note of in recent years?

MM: The gut has been very severely damaged by excessive use of antibiotics. People might say, "Well, I haven't had any antibiotics in years, so I'm fine." But ninety percent of the antibiotics used in this country are given to livestock. So, if you're eating nonorganic beef, chicken, turkey, or pork, you're getting those antibiotics through consuming those foods. It's a big problem that's destroying the gut. Excess sugar is also harmful to the gut. Food sensitivities destroy the lining of the gut and create intestinal permeability, which then allows larger molecules of food and toxins to get into the blood and cause inflammation. That's responsible for things like rheumatoid arthritis and different inflammatory conditions like eczema and psoriasis.

The gut is critical—and its healthy development in children begins at preconception. During pregnancy, moms should be eating cultured vegetables, natural organic yogurts without sugar, and taking a good probiotic. These are all ways that moms can lay a great foundation for her own microbiome. So when the child is ready to be exposed to the bacteria when they're passing through the birth canal, they too will benefit from that good friendly flora.

DB: You mentioned in your article, which I found very interesting, about pesticides being dangerous whether you're using them, consuming, or living in an area that sprays them as a high-risk factor for autism.

MM: Yes. They've done studies in California, where they show the closer pregnant women and children were to the spraying of pesticides the higher incidence of autism.

There are three billion pounds of pesticides sprayed on our crops each year. These are chemicals that were created during World War II to kill our enemies. When the war ended, scientists thought, "What are we to do with these chemicals?" They decided to spray them on crops and kill the insects or the weeds. People didn't realize that if they're killing insects and they're killing weeds, then they're eventually going to be problematic for the human body. They wreak havoc on our environmental and biological systems.

DB: Are there any types of supplements that you think a mother should talk to her child's pediatrician about if she already has a child on the spectrum?

MM: Definitely. We started a physician-training course as part of the Autism Research Institutes conferences because your average pediatrician didn't have the expertise to know what to give or how to help these kids. It is not part of their training. For example, they're not aware of the fact that many children on the autism spectrum who are very picky eaters, respond well and will broaden their food repertoire when given zinc in small incremental doses. When it's brought in gradually, it often results in the child becoming less picky.

That's usually done in combination with a whole host of other supplements and dietary changes. I'd love to say there's a magic bullet. If a mom just gives a child on the spectrum a good comprehensive multi with adequate B6, zinc, magnesium, omega-3 fatty acids, and a probiotic—and removes gluten, dairy, and sugar—that certainly would be a good step in the right direction.

DB: I find most people will wait until their child is diagnosed until they start trying to fix them. What advice would you give to parents on this subject?

MM: Well that is true for pretty much all conditions. It's changing now thankfully, but as Dr. Baker has said many times from the podium at various conferences, "People would rather die or change their religion before they change their diet." I think people tend to ignore early messages and wait too long to make changes to their diet and lifestyle.

The human body is amazing in that it sends us signals (usually mild ones at first) that tell us something is awry. If we would just listen and honor those early signals a little bit better, we could often prevent the full display or the full problem. Unfortunately, we don't. I used to work for a pathologist, Dr. Ali, who said when the body needs help, it gets together and elects a "spokes-organ." That spokes-organ might be your gut or your heart, liver, kidneys, etc. You're getting these signals, but then too often we take medicine to mask the symptoms instead of honoring those initial messages and making the appropriate changes necessary to prevent a full-blown illness.

DB: How important is prevention and maintenance? With my daughter, I was able to get rid of the eczema holistically and it's been gone a few years, but I still watch her closely and continue to put in all types of supplements and do testing for her. For me it's an ongoing process, given we live in such a toxic world.

MM: Food is medicine and food is the key to health. It's our responsibility as parents to learn as much as we can about healthy food and help our kids understand how important it is. We also need to pay attention to the signals that our children's bodies give us. If they're full of mucus, take dairy out since it is very mucus-forming. If their immune system is weak, then take sugar out as sugar decreases the efficiency of the immune system immensely.

DB: What about people who say it's too expensive to buy healthy food? What do you tell them?

MM: There are tricks to the trade and there are ways to minimize the time and expense. My husband and I weren't making that much money back when we were buying all organic food and making our own baby food. We found ways to make food in batches and freeze certain things.

Dr. Baker's famous saying that I believe he got from a Russian philosopher, "Follow those who seek the truth and flee from those who say they found it," is so true. Because we're all still learning—I don't have all the answers and I've been studying this stuff for thirty-eight years. Nobody has the answers for every single child, they are all different. As parents, we have to tune in and become aware that we're living in a toxic world, but there's so much we can do to minimize the damage of those toxins, starting with nutrition prior to conceiving, during pregnancy, and as our children grow.

✳ ✳ ✳

There are so many little things that you can do for your body to help it repair itself from the onslaught of toxins we are all exposed to each day. Some of these things include eating foods that we know detoxify the body, such as arugula and cilantro, to name a couple. Using organic spices can help keep the bad bacteria in your gut in check. Then you can also rotate supplements that will help get rid of your stored toxins. I will be speaking more about how to use food as medicine in the "My Kitchen" chapter as well as some of my favorite natural supplements in the "My Natural Medicine Cabinet" chapter later in the book.

I know Maureen gave you a lot to think about and it can feel overwhelming. I'm hoping to help by suggesting slight changes to your routine, such as dry cleaning at an organic dry cleaner, or incorporating more glass to use for food items instead of plastic. It's a good idea to switch out a few things that are easier and then build up to bigger items. Certainly, replacing toxic household cleaners with more eco-friendly ones is simple and not too costly. For some it may take a few months to notice a difference, but eventually you will feel revived.

My favorite part of Maureen's interviews is about the birthing process. Modern-day advances in medicine are important especially if you are in a car accident. However, when it comes to delivering a baby, medical practitioners seem to feel tremendous pressure to get your baby out quickly, even when it's not in your or the baby's best interest. I remember clearly how focused I was on giving birth naturally to my daughter and I had to fight so hard to make that happen.

Now that we have covered a lot of outside influences that affect the body's state of balance—whether they are food choices, use of plastic, or things from the environment thrust upon us—we will dig deeper into the biochemistry of autism and epigenetics. This way you will understand exactly why the lifestyle choices and ways to protect yourself from the environment are so vital for you to pay attention to. Everything we do affects our DNA. Genes can get turned on from things you choose to eat. Some of these genes are responsible for putting you at risk for Parkinson's or autism for example. Once you turn on a gene on it can be hard to turn it off. So again, prevention is always key to protect the delicate processes of the body.

CHAPTER SUMMARY

Take an inventory of all the personal care, cleaning, and laundry products that you use and replace them with healthier, less toxic versions.

Carefully take the time to write out your birth plan. Make sure to sit down with your OBGYN to go over it and consider asking her or him to sign it.

Stay away from genetically modified food and foods treated with hormones or pesticides.

Limit exposure to as many dangerous plastics and other hormone disrupting chemicals as you can.

Do things to promote the health of your microbiome before getting pregnant, such as taking probiotics, eating fermented food, and staying away from processed junk food.

Don't wait too long to get your child looked at if there are symptoms, as the damage goes deeper the longer you wait.

Remember, food is medicine.

Chapter 8

THE BIOCHEMISTRY OF AUTISM

with Scott Smith, PA

There are a host of changes that can occur on a cellular level due to stress, a less than optimal diet and exposure to environmental toxins long before an autism diagnosis is given. These outside influences can really add up and negatively impact your child's health, which is the reason we are going to dive deeper into the intricate cellular processes that go on inside the body to create imbalance and ultimately an illness. Many of these things of course cannot be seen by the naked eye for some time in the way of symptoms. For this reason, holistic practitioners will look for certain signs in blood work, urine, or stool tests that give them clues as to what might be going on in the body, especially if your child is experiencing any symptoms or would like to prevent a particular disease that has already taken hold of one family member, as in the case of my son.

Once you have experienced a full-fledged autoimmune or chronic illness, it is very easy to look back and see all the things that may have added up and contributed to your problem. I have no doubt now what my son's road map to autism looks like and the things we passed along the way to get to that dreaded diagnosis. Unfortunately, ten years later, most mainstream doctors still don't recognize any of the signs that he experienced. I am talking about the current pediatricians who, for instance, still think that having eczema, chronic ear infections, and constipation is all part of a normal childhood. Unfortunately, the truth is that these low-grade chronic conditions are making up the "new" normal and left alone each one of these symptoms could continue to fester and grow, possibly snowballing into something much bigger like asthma or autism eventually.

There is no doubt that I was hell bent on preventing autism in my daughter, however, I also did not want her to suffer from any of the other childhood chronic conditions either. I knew that I could achieve immune balance if I worked hard and just paid attention to what her body was telling me. And my daughter's body told me so many things, especially in those first few years. I really believe that one wrong turn could have had devastating consequences for us.

So even with everything I learned and studied from Dylan, it was still not smooth sailing for Jessica. As I mentioned in Chapter 3, she developed food allergies, eczema, and then later chronic constipation. We started searching for clues very early on. I was testing her vitamin D, B12, and her homocysteine levels very early in the first year. Next came the food allergy panels, which revealed her dairy allergy and sensitivities to other foods, which also showed that she had gut dysbiosis and permeability issues. I brought Jessica in for her first speech evaluation at nine months and it revealed that she was already experiencing a significant delay. Again, this was amazing information to have, just as much as it was incredibly upsetting. I knew that if I just had all the information earlier this time around that I could do something to prevent autism in my next child. And fortunately, I was absolutely right.

Then at eighteen months, the most devastating news I could possibly have received was that she had lead poisoning, which was detected in a test done by a specialty laboratory. This test looked at all her amino acids, neurotransmitter levels, and certain heavy metals. I couldn't wrap my head around why this was not detected six months prior at her twelve-month well-visit. But how alarmed would a regular doctor have been even if a level of eight was found, since anything under ten is still considered "normal." No level of lead should ever be considered safe or acceptable. Please do not let someone talk you into the idea that even a moderate level is fine.

I immediately took Jessica to the smartest practitioners I knew to help me get the lead out of her body safely before the whole situation snowballed into something really devastating. A friend of mine told me about a physician's assistant, Scott Smith who was really helping children with some of the more difficult-to-treat illnesses, or sometimes we refer to them as "slow responders." This is a term for a child that is so sick that no matter what you do, there can be very little change or progress for a long period of time.

A few years back, my son was considered to be a slow responder until we finally moved a boulder after chipping away at his health for many years. I will never forget how my friend described Scott. She said, "He is so smart and could definitely be teaching biochemistry to medical students." That's all I needed to hear and off I went to make an appointment for both of my kids. I got four opinions on how to handle Jessica's lead dilemma and I ended up going with Scott's suggestion to use oral vitamin C to chelate the lead. Thankfully that decision really paid off. We did fecal metals tests while we were using the vitamin C and noticed that a lot more metals were coming out of her than just the lead. Fecal metal tests can monitor how much and what kind of metals are coming out after the chelating drug, or in this case natural substance, is given. Most people don't know that vitamin C can chelate many unwanted things from the body such as plastic, pesticides, and heavy metals. Jessica immediately leapt forward after I started administering the oral vitamin C with no negative consequences. I continued to work with Scott on her eczema and leaky gut with some pretty positive results. I believe Scott's treatment plan for removing the heavy metals was very instrumental in why she does not have autism or any other childhood chronic illness. She was literally starting to slip away and he helped me bring her back to life.

Scott Smith is a physician assistant who has a practice in Central Florida treating both adults and children suffering from chronic illness. Scott has also written about biomedical interventions being used for treating autism in several publications, and he also presents on the subject both nationally and internationally.

DB: Do you think that autism is increasing?

SS: It's growing by leaps and bounds. There's no justification you could put on this genetically, so there's some other sort of environmental trigger that's making this number go up dramatically. I know that sometimes people will say that these people are getting diagnoses that used to go to some other diagnostic category, but honestly you can't find the other diagnostic category that's lost population to justify that.

DB: That's interesting. Do you think that children in general are sicker today than say a decade ago?

SS: Absolutely. You and I see this all the time, they're much more vulnerable. Environmental toxins are a little bit different. Genetic anomalies that were not a problem for our parents and our parents' parents have now become problematic in the environment as it's constituted today.

DB: Do you think autism can be prevented?

SS: I think that we now have a better understanding of a fair number of triggers. I don't know if I could ever tell you that you could bring your relative risk down to zero, but I do think there's some preventative actions you could take to decrease your risk factor, that's for sure.

DB: I'd like to talk to you about when a child hits bumps in the road, meaning recognizing early signs that something has gone awry and dealing with it before it snowballs. Do you think Jessica's lead poisoning was a good example of that?

SS: Absolutely. We talk a lot about mercury toxicity in kids with ASD, but the World Health Organization thinks that lead toxicity is much more of a problem for kids because it's more readily available. It's a sub hydra reactive metal, it can accumulate in our moms. We know the biochemistry for the moms is not that much different than the kids. So, this can be passed across the placenta and through breast milk in addition to environmental exposure after birth. There are a number of potential sources for lead. Lead is probably more closely linked to learning disability and ADHD than is mercury by the way.

DB: Can you tell me a little bit about the mom's body burden? Can she pass on toxins even if she was exposed to them before her pregnancy and not during it?

SS: I believe that is possible. We know that pregnancy and breastfeeding are high metabolic states so the moms turn over a lot of fat tissue. They turn over a lot of bone tissue, which mobilizes this lead or any other heavy metal. That heavy metal can cross the placenta and, because all these heavy metals are fat soluble, they can come out through breast milk. We've seen it. We've checked breast milk samples and we've found toxic breast milk.

DB: Tell me a little bit about the moms and what you were talking about the anomalies and not being able to detox the heavy metals.

SS: I think this goes back to what we know about methylation and trans-sulfuration. We know that glutathione irregularities in autism are very common. We actually find them with high frequency in the parents as well. Not as much consequence from the dad as he can't pass heavy metals, he can only pass the gene set but moms can actually pass the metals.

DB: Tell us about this gene set that you're talking about including the problem with glutathione. Some other practitioners have mentioned it.

SS: These are actually probably more of a genomic anomaly than they would be a full genetic break. This is where we talk about things like MTHFR, which is methylenetetrahydrofolate reductase. This is how you convert folic acid from your diet from eating green leafy vegetables and things like that or folic acid in the supplemental form. This is how you convert this into the tetrahydrofolate pool to eventually make methylfolate. We find that this MTHFR occurs at a higher frequency in kids with ASD and related disorders, and also in their family members, than it does in the general population.

DB: Do you find MTHFR to be an issue for children with autism or contributing to autism?

SS: Absolutely. A great article that was written by Dr. Jill James back in 2006. My office at the time was a collaborating contributor to that article. We found that there was a certain set of genomes that left kids at a higher vulnerability for ASD. MTHFR was probably the most dominant in that group. There was also some RFC, which is the reduce folate carrier. There was some COMT, which is catechol-O-methyltransferase. We keep adding to the list. Now we know that dihydrofolate reductase can become problematic. These are all genome tests that you can get and remediate. These are all things that can be made to work better. You can't correct a broken genome, but you can sure work around that break a little to make the biochemistry a bit more successful.

DB: What should someone who has not been exposed to any of these SNPs (single nucleotide polymorphisms) like, I have to know about MTHFR? What kinds of things can they do if they test for it and find they're positive?

SS: Methylfolate is the end product. This is what comes out of the MTHFR single nucleotide polymorphism. When we say SNP, that's what that means. Methylfolate is the product that's made there and this is what the body needs to complete the transaction. The body donates that methyl group from methylfolate to make the methylation pathway spin. You also need to make methylfolate to trigger a separate independent pathway called the tetrahydrobiopterin pathway, which is responsible for controlling your blood vessel diameter and nitric oxide synthase and all these other really cool things.

So, if you cut that off at the knees and your methylfolate content is low, you're missing the raw materials to make these very important pathways spin. Now they're left spinning using secondary or tertiary methyl donors, which are not nearly as efficient. Methylfolate is particularly useful in the brain. It concentrates in the brain four times higher than it concentrates in other body tissues. Often times when that methylfolate starts to fail you, the first place you see the symptoms is neurologically because the brain becomes depleted much faster, because the usage of methylfolate is so great.

DB: Would this have to do with the ability to detox well?

SS: Absolutely yes. If you saw that biochemistry down the pathway, like the Plinko game on *The Price Is Right*, the end point of this pathway is to make cysteine and glutathione. These are what we call sulfation molecules. When you want to take a fat-soluble toxin like lead or mercury or organophosphates and pesticides and all these other things, you have to make them water-soluble to clear them. One of the primary ways that you would take something from fat-soluble to water-soluble is to sulfate it. Cysteine and glutathione are your sulfur donators so if you don't make those well, all of a sudden a lot of these fat-soluble toxins are going to be stored in the body and not be able to be cleared.

DB: Can you tell me a little bit more about the biochemistry of autism? A lot of people think of it as a psychological disorder and this example above is just one component of how the immune system goes off track. What do you think are the highlights of the biochemistry with autism that are important for people who wouldn't know anything about it because they haven't experienced it yet? Please tell us a little bit about it.

SS: I try to follow a pretty simple biomarker-based approach. I think that there are three key areas that you have to have a good understanding in for every kid to have a successful biomedical plan. You have to have a good understanding of that methylation pathway that includes the folic acid cycle, methylation, and transsulfation. You have to have a good understanding of the mitochondria and you have to have a good understanding of what is going on in the GI tract. We find a lot of research now is coming out about how broken our GI tracts are in our kids with ASD that they have abnormal flora, permeability issues, and immune system dysregulation in the GI tract.

A number of studies have come out to help support that claim. My initial investigation into kids is to look at those three areas, have a good understanding of what's going on and fix as much of it as we can before we even start looking outside that box. They're a little bit more closely linked together than people give them credit for. Even though I consider them three separate entities, there's a lot of overlap. For example, if your methylation pathway is broken, you do not make a product called SAMe. SAMe is your universal methyl donor, and without it you can't repair DNA, RNA, and cell membranes. You can't clear neurotransmitters properly. You can't make glutathione properly and you can't protect your mitochondria.

A lot of times what I find is our kids start off life with a kink in that methylation ability and as the toxins build up and the methylation pathway can't do what it's supposed to do. All of a sudden your mitochondria, immune system, and your GI tract become a bit suspect. The earlier in life you can identify some of these anomalies, in particular on that methylation pathway, you can prevent a lot of this stuff from snowballing downhill.

DB: Tell us a little bit about the mitochondria issues that people would need to understand.

SS: For a long time, people thought that you were either born with a good set of mitochondria or you were born with a bad set of mitochondria and there was just nothing you could do about it. That was proven to be untrue in the late 2000s. We started to look at mitochondria as something that you could actually damage after birth, that you could actually have an acquired damage to mitochondria. Every cell has mitochondria by the way. Each mitochondrion has five complexes. They each do a little bit of a different job, and they're linked together like pearls on a necklace by something called the electron transport chain. Dr. Richard

Kelley at Kennedy Krieger found that in ASD, in particular regressive ASD, that complex 1 was very vulnerable. Complex 1 is vulnerable to a toxic exposure, to oxidative damage or inflammatory response.

This damage has been found to occur in our kids with ASD. The good news about complex 1 anomalies is that you can actually make complex 1 work pretty good. If you find it broken, there are things you can do nutritionally and biomedically to make that complex work much better, such as control oxidative stress by making glutathione levels rise, taking care of any toxicity burden that a child may have, and then providing nutritional support to facilitate improved complex 1. This includes carnitine, CoQ10, B vitamins, and creatine. There is a whole list of them. We collectively call these things mitochondria cocktails, and each kid's cocktail is a little bit different depending on their particular needs.

DB: I'm going to talk about Jessica, since she is a great example of someone whose mitochondria got damaged after birth because of the lead poisoning. Then she had the gross motor issues and later the strabismus. Can you talk a little bit about how a child may not have autism, but show soft signs of some mitochondria damage?

SS: Again, mitochondria are in every cell in the human body. We start thinking mitochondria in the general population when you have anomalies going on in more than one organ system that don't seem to be tied together. For our kids, it's a little bit different because the toxicity exposure is universal so all the cells could be affected. You could get muscular involvement, which could lead to some hypotonia, causing things like strabismus where one of the eye muscles is stronger than the other. You can get neurocognitive problems where attention, focus, and neurologic development could become problematic. We can see it in a number of ways.

DB: Let's talk about that third component, which is the gut.

SS: This is where I think the rubber meets the road for a lot of our kids. A paper came out by Dr. Richard Frye and Dr. Derrick MacFabe in the last couple of years showing how these can overlap. It showed that the toxin produced by clostridia species can also facilitate damage to complex 1 and affect the mitochondria. The toxic exposure doesn't necessarily have to be lead, as in the case of Jessica, or mercury like we think for some of our kids. It could actually be something growing in the GI tract. So, controlling the microbiota in the large and the small intestine are important for our children. Our kids often have immune system problems and are often on frequent antibiotics. We have a lot of babies born by C-section, which affects the normal development of microbiota. We have some kids who don't tolerate milk, including breast milk. These are all things that can set you up for abnormal flora in the GI tract.

Add to that, I believe a lot of our kids suffer from some hypochlorhydria, which means not making enough stomach acid. Some of our kids suffer from pancreatic insufficiency where they don't make enough digestive enzymes. Our kids often have motility problems where they are either constipated or have some diarrhea. All these things will lead to flora changes in the GI tract. All the pathogenic bacteria that we talk about in our kids, these are all opportunistic infections. They're not exposed to these bacteria more than say you or I, Dara, in some kids there is better opportunity for them to grow so they become the dominant species.

DB: Is this similar to the mitochondria in that there are preventative measures one can take to help the person become more balanced?

SS: For sure. So, once you've identified that you have a problem, the problem could be weight loss, poor appetite, or night waking (and it's not always a direct GI symptom), but once you identify that you've got some abnormal flora, then you can figure out a way to target it. Primarily, we would look for yeast species populations overgrowing. We would look for clostridia-type bacteria overgrowing. Then I also take a look for gram-negative bacteria. Gram-negative bacteria in their cell wall have something called lipopolysaccharide. So, if this lipopolysaccharide is able to get through a damaged GI tract, it's one of the more inflammatory things that we know of to the human immune system and to the nervous system. There's a number of animal studies that actually show that lipopolysaccharide from a GI source can cause microglia activation in the brain, which is something that our kids struggle with as well.

DB: How would someone test for these three things? And should they test for them especially if they have another sibling on the spectrum already?

SS: The beauty of some of this testing is it's not invasive. You can get a good representation of what's going on very early in life without requiring a blood draw. You can do stool testing. You can do urine samples in the form of an organic acid test and these give you predictive markers for overgrowth. You would also look for traditional GI symptoms: constipation or diarrhea, bloated belly (particularly those kids whose bellies start out pretty flat in the beginning of the day and as the day goes on they get really distended), excessive reflux as a baby, spitting up—things like that. Those would be all things that you could look for. Changing around some probiotics, changing around some dietary strategies, avoiding medications that block stomach acid would all be key to helping heal up that GI tract. Antibiotics can be used for a short-term benefit. You use the antibiotics to get acute control and then we set up protocols to help repair and stabilize the flora.

DB: How would you test in the other two areas?

SS: Let's start with genomic anomalies in methylation in particular. For kids who can complete this type of test, you could get a 23andMe profile, which is available online without a prescription. It is a saliva sample so it's a little difficult to get on the younger kids, but if you get that, it will send you raw data. That raw data then can be fed into another website called Genetic Genie. They'll give you a methylation breakdown and a detoxification breakdown. And it will give you all the gene SNPs on that methylation transsulfation pathway. It costs you about $100 to $110 total to get all that done.

        MTHFR can be done as a blood test. It's a simple test, it can be done through LabCorp or Quest, but not every insurance will cover these genetic tests so in that fashion it can be a little expensive. The test can cost up near four-hundred dollars without any insurance coverage, so you want to make sure that your insurance will cover it before you request a test. There are some other profiles you can get with some SNPs. I believe Great Plains and Doctor's Data offer some testing as well that are blood drawn. Once I know the genetics, I like to get an additional profile called methylation pathway that we send off to Amsterdam, which actually gives us the functional status of that pathway right then and there. The genomics are great; it gives you a predictive value of how that pathway is probably working. But it's always great to see in real time how the functional testing matches up with the genomic testing.

Then for the mitochondria, that one is going to probably be best achieved using blood testing. We get a certain level of test for kids that we suspect with mitochondria dysfunction and under a certain physiologic condition. I like to draw my mitochondria testing, at least my first line testing, after a three-hour fasting period. I prefer it not be a full overnight fast because we look at an amino acid profile and even if the individual amino acids are normal, it's the ratio of certain amino acids to other amino acids.

DB: Do you find that some of your clients are doing this as a preventative test? If so, has it been a positive experience for them?

SS: Actually, a lot of people have done it with great success, including yourself, not only in the siblings but in the parents. They are following some of these protocols and feeling much better. Parents who didn't necessarily feel poorly, we identify some of this stuff and we start to correct it. And then they feel better. They realize where their actual deficits were, so it helps out tremendously. Besides siblings and parents, we've even crossed over and looked at cousins, aunts, and uncles when they had similar enough symptoms to make sure that there weren't problems in other families too. By just learning the methylation, mitochondria and microbiota status from the one child with ASD, it can benefit several family members simultaneously.

DB: Do you find that a pretty good size of the population has a problem with at least one of these three areas?

SS: I think that abnormalities in any one of these three areas for almost any person probably would leave them vulnerable. Now we're linking increased gut permeability and abnormal flora as a potential trigger for autoimmunity, allergies, and atopic dermatitis, mitochondria insufficiency, chronic fatigue, and fibromyalgia. Methylation defects can go across the board, but for middle-aged men, methylation defects can lead to hyperhomocysteinemia and have cardiac complications. MTHFR and methylation defects have been linked with migraine with aura and miscarriages in women. It goes well beyond ASD.

DB: Were you surprised how quickly Jessica got better on your vitamin C protocol to get the metals out?

SS: Not at all, because if you think about what we did for her, we were using vitamin C as our chelating agent, which was very well described by Dr. Boyd Haley several years ago. In addition to helping her detoxify, the vitamin C is a phenomenal antioxidant so in one fell swoop we took off two pressure points from complex 1 and mitochondria. We took out toxicity and oxidative stress from being problems and her mitochondria started working better. Not only did we detoxify her, but we improved mitochondria status with one type of treatment.

DB: That treatment was such a success for her.

SS: Every time I saw her she looked better than the previous time.

DB: She's still doing all her supplements from her protocol. I don't stop them just because she is doing better. That actually brings me to a question that I have. Do you think it's really important for children, given how toxic the world is today, to have some sort of prevention and maintenance program, even if they get themselves over some kind of chronic issue as Jessica did?

SS: The world is a much more toxic place than when we grew up or our parents grew up. In addition to heavy metal exposures, we now have many more endocrine disruptors. We have more genetically modified and overly processed food. Our kids are not getting the nutritional support that they once got, and their GI tracts are breaking down at a very early time. They're becoming toxic at a very early age. In addition to ASD numbers rising, there are increases in ADHD and learning disabilities. I suspect that they probably all have a very similar starting point to autism.

DB: Do you think it's a lot easier to treat someone who has some soft signs such as food allergies or eczema rather than trying to bring someone back from autism?

SS: I would never say that we have treatments for autism per se, but we identify all these underlying factors. If we can get them early enough, they're not as deep seated. And it doesn't take as much time for them to recover and there's not as much damage done.

If you can identify these symptoms when they're very young, it can make a difference especially in the siblings. The parents do have an acute awareness and they become very keen to even mild changes in their children after they've already had one child with ASD (autism spectrum disorder). We're picking those kids up at ten months, twelve months, or fifteen months. We start some biomedical treatment programs and stop progression with additional symptoms.

DB: I've talked to some practitioners who say that they find that it's harder to recover a child today than let's say ten years ago just because the world is a little bit more toxic and the food supply is different. Do you find that's true for you?

SS: I don't know if it's more difficult, but it's definitely different. What we did to help kids in the early 2000s is not the same way that we would do to take care of kids today. Again, there are more toxicity and endocrine disruptors. We know way more now, so back in the early 2000s, we only had a couple of tools in our toolbox and now we have multiple tools. We also have multiple things that we have to check. So, any given time, when you're doing a comprehensive biomedical treatment program, you could be managing GI tract anomalies. You could be dealing with methylation defects. You're going to be dealing with toxicity issues. You might be dealing with immune system dysfunction. You might be dealing with a thyroid problem. Now I find that the kids have many more breaks that you have to fix. It looks a little different and the treatment is a little different. I don't know if it's more difficult, it's just different.

DB: Let's talk about these early signs or, as we call them, "soft signs." For instance, many times when a child has eczema it's not taken seriously since it's considered so common. Everybody thinks it's no big deal. But to me, when Jessica had eczema it meant her immune system was totally off kilter, which could have snowballed into something more serious. Can you talk a little bit about why it's important to recognize some of these softer chronic illnesses like eczema or food allergies and try to nip them in the bud?

SS: Just like you're saying, Dara, we're not just looking for the early signs of autism. We're looking for those one-off symptoms. We're looking for a kid who has excessive spitting up, is intolerant to milk at an early age, develops eczemas, or atypical rashes, kids that are not good sleepers with night waking.

Often times what we find in the siblings is that there's atypical rashes, intolerance to foods, maybe bloated belly, constipation, and diarrhea, just things that you wouldn't expect to come across. These parents have again a keen eye, and they're like, "Oh jeez, this is abnormal. Every time we give little Johnny milk, he has projectile vomiting." Even though he doesn't necessarily test as a classic IgE allergy to milk, we might have something else going on here."

DB: Do you think of autism as autoimmune?

SS: I think that for some children autoimmunity does play a role. A broad concept that I like to use is that I think that the immune system is working against the body. It's not necessarily making autoimmune reactions, but sometimes the immune system gets primed in a way that it makes exaggerated immune responses to things it's not supposed to. That's atypical or a reaction to foods that should not become problematic. The immune system dysfunction in our kids is real. There's a certain subset with autoimmunity, but for more of the kids I think a better descriptive term would be immune system dysfunction. The immune system is just not behaving right.

DB: Do you find that prevention is multifaceted? Should parents understand that you have to do more than just one thing?

SS: Yes, it would be so much easier if we could just concentrate on one thing. If that was the case, I think that the number of cases of ASD, learning disability, and ADHD would go down dramatically. The problem is that it is multifactorial and not every kid has the exact same symptoms. What one sibling has may not be the same symptoms that another sibling has in the same family. You have to be aware of all of these different symptoms. Like you're saying, allergies, atopic dermatitis, eczema, sleeping problems, and GI tract problems, those should all be triggers that you're sitting on a potential powder keg and that you would want to fix them before it became problematic.

DB: What could something like eczema or one of these other conditions you've just mentioned fester and become if they were to all of a sudden get hit with a couple more problems such as toxins?

SS: I think that eczema already tells you that you're a little bit imbalanced with that immune system. You're keeping your body healthy using what's called a T-helper 2 response, which is a much more inflammatory response. Any other things that you add onto that that are T-helper 2 stimulants like a toxic exposure, certain viruses, things like that will push you further and further and create more and more symptoms as time goes on. You'd want to be really careful with a kid who presented with the classic signs of atopy, which would be eczema, asthma, food allergies, or seasonal allergies.

DB: Who should consider getting some testing done on their baby or on themselves? Would it be concerning if a pregnant woman has some things that run in her family especially if they are autoimmune by nature?

SS: Obviously if you already have a child who has some developmental delay, autism spectrum disorder, then I think that you would want to test immediately before you had another baby so you could try to remediate as much as you could in the parents and have a good starting point for treatment as soon as the baby is born.

　　For people who are expecting their first child or want to have their first child, there are a few things that we think are worthwhile to look at in moms in particular. I think to know the MTHFR status would be phenomenal. I believe looking at your thyroid function is important. We know that moms with poor thyroid function during pregnancy have a higher rate of having kids with ASD or ADHD. You'd want to take a look at free fatty acid status as well. MTHFR, free fatty acid, and thyroid function would be a general basic starting points I think that anyone who was concerned and wanted to take all the preventative steps that they possibly could would take a look at.

DB: How important is diet and nutrition for prevention?

SS: Your diet is your greatest food source, so we use those nutrients to protect ourselves, to heal up damaged tissue. If you're not feeding the body the appropriate nutrients not only can it create damage, but it doesn't allow you to go back and repair damage that's already occurred.

When I take a look at some of these kids now and they open up their lunch box and they've got a bottle of Ensure and a baggy full of Goldfish crackers or maybe a Lunchable, it makes me shudder. I'm not quite sure how these kids will make it through life without any complications with diets like that. Eventually it will come back to bite them in the backside.

DB: Are there any supplements that you think are very important for parents to consider giving their baby or child?

SS: I think that there are three supplements that just about every kid in the United States probably deserves to be on in some way shape or form. I think just a basic good quality multivitamin, which I don't think any pediatrician would argue. I think our kids should be on an omega-3 fatty acid supplement. I think that the way that our diet is overly processed, we've gotten away from a fish-based diet. You really shouldn't eat a lot of fish anyway because of contamination. You want to make sure that it's been molecularly distilled, so that toxins have been removed. I do think that you should also have your children on a basic probiotic.

DB: The last area I wanted to talk about is what might be driving this immense increase. There are a lot of theories out there, a lot of different things that might be contributors. In my case, I look back at Dylan and his perfect storm. I can think of like twenty-five things. I'm just hoping that you could share what could be going on. It doesn't necessarily have to be your opinion. What are people talking about, other colleagues and professionals. What are some general things that we're not sure that could be contributors to chronic illness in general and autism?

SS: Like you were saying with Dylan, the things you can look back now and you identify are so numerous. You're like, "Oh my gosh. No wonder this happened." I do think that changes in our diet and changes in stress levels. We have a much more stressed mom getting pregnant nowadays. They're probably bringing children to stressful situations. I don't want to hammer on vaccinations, but I do think vaccinations are a potential trigger. We know that using acetaminophen has been linked in a number of studies to increasing your risk factor. Acetaminophen stops your body from producing glutathione for a short period of time after a single dose. We're using Roundup on our lawns. The endocrine disruptors are a big problem too. We are exposed to phthalates from drinking bottled water much more than we did a couple of generations ago. So, diet, toxic exposures, whether it be from vaccinations or from poor dietary choices or other environmental exposures, I think those are our big keys.

DB: In many instances a friend tells someone to call me because maybe the husband has ADD and he's concerned about having a child with autism. Are there any conditions that parents might have whether it's colitis or ADD, where they might pay special attention to the information in this book, rather than someone who has no chronic illness and no other child on the spectrum?

SS: Yes, absolutely. In particular, we would worry about family history of any autoimmune disease. One of the questions I ask all families when they come is if there has been any family history of autoimmune disease. I do think that increases your risk factor a little bit.

DB: Is it common when you look back to find children who are diagnosed with autism to have a mom that was suffering from an illness while pregnant? When I talk to women that I meet in the autism community, many of them had something such as Hashimoto's, fibromyalgia, or in my case, multiple chemical sensitivities. I think people don't realize if they're sick that it's going to have an effect on their baby.

SS: Again, we're not trying to point fingers at anybody, but there are usually some things going on behind the scenes, more often with mom than with dad, but dads don't get off one-hundred-percent scott-free here. When we go back and start picking through mom's history, it's not uncommon to find something of concern.

DB: I guess the last thing we want to do is leave parents on a positive note. We obviously cannot control everything. But do you think if we tried to be extra cautious with as much as we possibly can, including more natural personal care and cleaning products, organic food, and stay away from pesticides, that we can really decrease our risk? Do you think that parents have a much greater chance of having a child without chronic illness and especially autism if they do these things we have outlined in the book and specifically this chapter?

SS: Yes, we've actually seen it time and time again. There's no guarantee because there are factors that we probably don't even understand or know exist yet. I think if we can control what we can—like diet, chemical exposure, and pesticides—then your chance of a good outcome is pretty high.

✳ ✳ ✳

Again, parental autoimmune conditions greatly affect the health of their child. It's about changing what you can and supporting areas of the body that may be affected by the things you can't control. I feel as though we have to detox our bodies daily to some degree in order to stay healthy. You might think that sounds depressing, but I am happy to live my life paying attention to what I eat and the things I surround myself with. It helps me feel good and keep my family safe, and I hope it will do the same for you.

The most important takeaway from this chapter is that you can still turn things around once you recognize the early symptoms or soft signs. You can begin healing just by making some important changes to the food choices that you make each day. If only I could go back in time and do it all over again.

I will never forget one night I was out with a group of friends and one person was talking about her child's asthma. I mentioned that she should try taking dairy out since many times it can cause or exacerbate asthma. She looked at me, smiled and said, "That would be too hard." I looked back directly into her eyes and thought, "What could be harder than the possibility that your child could die from an asthma attack on the way to the hospital?" Then she smiled at me in an uncomfortable way and said that she would think about it.

Personally, I can't imagine what convenience or routine could be worth getting in the way of your child experiencing good health and enjoying their childhood. For me there is nothing. I continue to unturn every stone to help restore Dylan's health by reading and studying information for hours a day. My husband often makes fun of me that I read studies on PubMed for fun while I am eating lunch. But you don't have to be as passionate or obsessed as I am to make a really significant difference for you or your child. Just implementing some simple steps and changes in your life can ultimately have a huge impact.

Please consider giving yourself and family this beautiful gift. I doubt you will ever regret trying but it's possible you may regret not doing something.

CHAPTER SUMMARY:

Your mitochondria can be damaged after birth by toxins.

You can test for genetic anomalies that may increase the chance of a child developing autism. If they are positive for any of these SNPs, then there are ways to make the pathway work better such as using specific supplements.

A parent suffering from an autoimmune illness may have a higher risk of their child developing a chronic illness.

Soft signs should be looked at and recognized as early as possible. There are steps that one can take to remediate the situation before a chronic illness develops and the damage gets deeply seated.

Problems in one of the three areas of concern may put you at higher risk for developing an autoimmune disease and those are in the GI tract, mitochondria, and methylation. You can do testing to find out if you have a problem in any of these areas.

Mothers can pass on toxins through their breast milk.

There are a lot more negative outside influences today that can put your child at risk including eating GMO and overly processed food, exposure to pesticides, and endocrine disrupters.

Chapter 9

EPIGENETICS AND METABOLIC PATHWAYS
with Anju Usman, MD

The essence of this chapter is an extremely important concept: that we can do much to protect our health. Unfortunately, people have been convinced for years that our genes dictate everything and that nothing we do to try to protect our health will matter. This of course could not be further from the truth. Yes, we all have genes that will predispose us to certain illnesses, which is where the phrase "runs in my family" comes from, but for the most part our personal choices make a big difference on whether or not we will develop a particular disease. This has to do with the study of epigenetics, which is a fast-growing field in the study of medicine. Please keep in mind that this does not apply to those conditions, which are considered genetic in basis, such as Down syndrome or fragile X—these are chromosomal aberrations as opposed to auto-immunity. I am referring to all the acquired chronic illnesses.

Autism is one condition that some professionals will say you are born with. However, more than 90 percent of the cases of autism are diagnosed as regressive autism, which means the child was developing normally and then they lost certain skills. Experts in the field have explained over and over that there is no such thing as a genetic epidemic, so it must be linked to environmental influences. We have gone over many of these outside influences such as mother's body burden, compromised microbiome at birth, antibiotic use, pesticides, heavy metal exposure, and vaccines. Each of these can wreak havoc on their own and the synergistic effect of them combined can prove to be too much, as explained by many professionals as the total load theory.

So even though genes are not solely to blame for this epidemic of autism, it does not mean that their expression does not influence how our bodies react in the face of environmental stressors. Two children from different families with the exact same environmental stressors may develop different chronic conditions, and some children in that same situation are unaffected. This is where gene expression comes into play. We have touched on one genetic variation in particular that can make children more vulnerable to developing autism in that it impairs our detoxification system.

In this chapter, we are going to learn a little bit more about the importance of metabolic pathways and what it means when they are not working at full capacity due to the presence of these genetic variations that block a particular pathway. Scott already touched on this in the previous chapter. Next we will explore how one can support the pathways to make them more efficient. There are many genetic variations that can put you at higher risk for specific conditions, but we will focus on the ones most closely associated with autism. Each one of my family members has two copies of a couple of these genetic variations that we will be exploring. The one that my son and I have two copies of puts us at high risk for both autism and Alzheimer's. As you can see this information is helpful to both parent and child.

I know of at least three of my father's siblings who suffered from Alzheimer's, which I always refer to as the adult form of autism. Someone once made an interesting comment to me that the person who was born seventy years ago develops Alzheimer's while the child born today with those same genes gets autism. I wholeheartedly believe that you can change the course of your family history or what you think it's supposed to be by making simple lifestyle choices to things in your diet and environment. Your genes do not ultimately have to dictate what will happen to you.

I have chosen a very knowledgeable doctor who is extremely passionate about this subject and can speak to it on a personal level as well. Dr. Anju Usman devotes her private practice to treating children with autism and other chronic health issues. She speaks nationally at conferences to help educate parents and practitioners, as well as researching various important topics as they relate to complex children's conditions. Dr. Usman holds a medical degree from Indiana University and is board certified in family practice as well as integrative and holistic medicine. She sits on the board and is involved in many well-known autism organizations including Generation Rescue, TACA (Talk About Curing Autism), and the Autism Society of Illinois. Dr. Usman also founded PURE Compounding Pharmacy that produces medicine for children who are sensitive or have serious allergies.

DB: What are your thoughts on whether autism is increasing?

AU: I do think autism is increasing. The numbers have shown that. The statistics have shown that autism has gone from one in ten thousand when I was in medical school in the late 1980s, to now one in forty-five. If you think about that rise, that's not just better diagnosis—so what is actually going on? The term epidemic has come up a lot and it does seem that with the rise in numbers that there is an epidemic of children being diagnosed with autism. And there's no such thing as a genetic epidemic, so there is something going on in our environment with what's happening to our children.

DB: Do you think children in general are sicker today?

AU: It's not just autism. There is an epidemic of childhood cancer. There's an epidemic of childhood allergies, asthma, and autoimmune issues as well. The statistics are alarming. One out of ten children are also now diagnosed with ADD and the question arises: what's happening to our kids and why are they so sick?

DB: Do you think that the risks of autism can be minimized and prevented in some situations?

AU: Absolutely. Again, if we don't think that this is a genetic disorder and we've not been able to prove that. We find with the whole human genome being studied and looking for the autism gene, that there isn't such a gene. So, if this is not a genetic condition there's something happening epigenetically.

DB: What does that term mean, "epigenetically?"

AU: Epigenetics is a fancy term for how our environment interplays with our genes. So, we might have genetic predispositions. Our parents, grandparents, and our ancestors might have certain predispositions to what we see in autism as autoimmunity or immune issues. If we know about those genetic predispositions, then we might be able to adjust our environment to prevent those genetics from being expressed. That's the whole concept around epigenetics, the interplay between the environment and our genes, whether genes can be turned on or turned off. It's very hard to turn it off, so to keep these genes that really shouldn't be expressed from being expressed is kind of the key.

DB: What types of things help prevent autism or greatly minimize the risk?

AU: When you're talking about autism, and we can't figure out a cause, what you have to look at is multiple factors and issues that might be creating this spectrum of disorders that we call autism. You have to look at what are the possible causes and our focus then gets turned to this whole concept of epigenetics in the environment and what could be triggering the immune system to show what we see metabolically in these kids.

   Prevention is going to be very broad in this case; looking at diet, nutrition, and the environment using what we call the precautionary principle. The precautionary principle essentially states that when you don't know what's going on and you're faced with this type of epidemic, you use precautions to prevent what you think might be happening even though we may not have all the science and all the clinical research to back us up at this time.

DB: If you could walk us through the common scenario that unfortunately you see often in your patients that develop autism.

AU: Mothers whose children go on to develop autism often tell me that their child experienced a normal pregnancy and delivery. The baby came home from the hospital and things were fine for a while, but eventually an increasing number of symptoms arose. Things like eczema, which is a potential allergic irritation on the skin that causes dermatitis and dryness. Even something like a history of colic and difficulty with formulas. Perhaps they weren't breastfed or they were born by C-section. And because of the C-section, they didn't receive that good bacteria during the delivery process that then seeds the gut lining and that good bacteria creates a really healthy immune system.

   The diversity of bacteria, the number of bacteria, the type of bacteria and yeast, and potentially good protozoa or parasites all make up our biome. A healthy biome is the key to developing a normal immune response and developing what we call healthy gut-brain connection. This gut-brain connection is a bidirectional communication network between the gut and the brain and vice versa. When a mom has C-section for example, the infant does not get exposed to the vaginal biome that goes on to seed the infants gastrointestinal tract. In vaginal births, the babies are inoculated with the good bacteria from vaginal and fecal material. Again, this good flora sets the stage for a healthy immune system. So, the question is if you do have a C-section, what can be done to provide your newborn with the good flora your child needs? I cannot tell you I've seen studies on this yet, but there are more practices and doctors who understand some of this, they're trying to get some of the vaginal secretions, some of the fecal secretions close to the child's face and nose to help inoculate the mucous membranes in the C-section delivered baby.

Again, from the get-go, if the mom has had a C-section or didn't nurse the baby, we may be setting the stage for an unhealthy or imbalanced immune system, and then that all too often leads to immune issues, like colic, eczema, or allergies. Then when we start feeding these susceptible infants foods that create inflammation like dairy products or gluten-containing foods like wheat. Then they start getting ear infections and congestion and are placed on antibiotics. This further depletes that microbiome and creates a lack of diversity in the bacteria of the child's body, and further weakens the immune system.

DB: How common is this?

AU: I hear this situation over and over again that, "My child was fine at their twelve-month birthday." They have great videos of them smiling, babbling, saying a few words and then by fifteen to eighteen months parents report a regression. The families tell me the child lost language and the ability to maintain eye contact. The history I get is that the parents say that they just lost the child they had. And that's so sad to hear because when we go back in the history parents will say hindsight is twenty-twenty; they can see that progression occurring and they didn't really understand what was happening or pay attention to it at the time. It's that burden of little things over time that accumulate and affect the immune system.

DB: When I go back in time I can see the same progression that you just spoke about with my own son. You look at his pediatric file, it's all there, everything you just mentioned: the food allergies, eczema, and the yeast rash. So, tell parents what should they do, keeping in mind the use of the precautionary principle if they start seeing some of these early signs that we've been talking about?

AU: The number one thing I would tell parents is listen to your intuition because a lot of parents know these things in their heart and they go to their pediatrician or they go to their doctor and the doctor says to them, "No, your child's fine. Don't worry. Everything's going to be okay." I'm not telling parents to worry or to distrust their pediatrician, but I am telling them that when they feel something is off, then they need to pay closer attention to that and not second-guess themselves.

I have four children and the same type of thing happened with my kids and I really didn't see it. I have pictures of my oldest daughter when she was about six months old and she's smiling, and in the background of the picture you can see her tongue completely covered in white. I know sometimes babies will drink formula and their tongue will be white, but this was the kind of white on the tongue that you cannot scrape off, called thrush. And thrush is a symptom of yeast overgrowth. Yeast really shouldn't be overgrown in our mouth, microbiome, or our GI tract because it prevents the healthy bacteria from growing. If we don't have good bacteria in our gut, then we can't develop our immune system properly when we are toddlers. Frequent diaper rashes that doesn't resolve is another sign of chronic yeast in the GI tract. I think issues such as eczema, food sensitivities, GI issues, chronic diaper rash, frequent infection are the big early warning signs that the immune system is starting to falter, and when antibiotics are introduced on top of that, it's basically a recipe for disaster.

Here is a chart that I compiled of all the early signs that each of the practitioners have mentioned. Please use it as a general reference. It should not be construed as a diagnosis of any illness.

EARLY WARNING SIGNS

SOFT SIGNS	ADVANCED SIGNS
Jaundice	Loss of Eye Contact
Colic	Loss of Language
Reflux	Constant Lining Up or Spinning Objects
Excessive Spitting Up	Stimming
Chronic Constipation	No Reciprocity

Multiple Food Allergies	Loss of Fine Motor Skills
Thrush	Loss of Gross Motor Skills
Chronic Diaper Rash	Inability to Chew or Swallow Food
Persistent Yeast or Fungal Rash	Inability to Crawl
Chronic Ear Infections	Extremely Late Crawling or Walking
Toe Walking	Perseverative Behaviors
Picky Eating	Child Not Developing Language at All

DB: What types of things can someone do once they notice these signs of possible yeast overgrowth or gut dysbiosis?

AU: Probably the most important thing would be to expose the child to good bacteria. I know that sounds kind of crazy, but in our society we are almost *too* hygienic. We don't get exposed to dirt. We don't get exposed to bacteria that we need to get exposed to in order to help develop a good immune system. We're too sterile. Parents can avoid things like antibacterial soaps and allow the child to share some of their good bacteria hopefully through touching and kissing. When we didn't have refrigeration, we used to ferment a lot of our foods to prevent them from going bad and culturing a lot of our foods. So, fermented foods and cultured foods are again, part of our tradition that helps our immune system to develop in a proper way.

A lot of people recommend probiotics, a supplement that is another way of getting some of that good bacteria in the gut, but with a small child I would recommend the foods that are from that child's heritage or ancestry; different cultures have adapted to respond well to different kinds of fermented foods. And then vitamin D is another really important vitamin that helps the immune system. What they're finding is that when women are vitamin D deficient in prepregnancy they are more likely to have a child with developmental delays. So, knowing your vitamin D status before you get pregnant and making sure your vitamin D status is good while you're pregnant is important, so that you can pass on that good vitamin D status to your child as well. Then getting your child plenty of vitamin D, which means sunshine, so that they don't become vitamin D deficient. Probiotics and vitamin D are probably the big two supplements that I use in my practice that help modulate the immune system the most.

DB: Could you tell us how to get the vitamin D tested and what level you feel it should be at for a woman who wants to get pregnant?

AU: The test to get a vitamin D level is vitamin D 25-OH or vitamin D 25-hydroxy. The reference range is usually thirty to one hundred and if you've got a child with developmental delays we probably want to see your vitamin D 25-hydroxy level closer to seventy. So, closer to that higher range, since we don't want it to be near thirty.

DB: I also noticed in your article on preventing autism that you talked about getting the thyroid and the copper-zinc ratio tested. You explain that this is important especially if you already have a child on the spectrum. Could you tell us about the importance of this copper-zinc ratio?

AU: The two important tests to have while you're pregnant or even before pregnancy is a zinc plasma level and a serum copper level and we want the ratios of those two tests to be one to one. Copper naturally increases during pregnancy. Copper is really important for angiogenesis of the placenta, so that means basically growing the placenta in a healthy fashion. We need plenty of copper during pregnancy.

What we find with copper is that it tends not to be an issue in terms of copper deficiency. In fact, it's the opposite since zinc tends to be deficient. Some women start off the pregnancy with low zinc. If copper-zinc ratio starts to widen during the pregnancy and if it becomes too wide, then at delivery the body has a big burden of copper because there is not enough zinc to balance it. What I see clinically is postpartum depression.

DB: That is very interesting.

AU: If we start the pregnancy with a fair amount of zinc, then we can prevent that imbalance between zinc and copper. Zinc is really important for the immune system as I mentioned before, it is also important for language, growth, and digestion. And it is also crucial for detoxification. If zinc is deficient in the mom, I would worry that it may be deficient in the newborn and that might again set that stage for the immune system to be challenged. I recommend pregnant women getting a copper-zinc ratio and trying to maintain a good balance of copper and zinc during their pregnancy in a one to one ratio.

DB: Why is it especially important for women to get their thyroid tested?

AU: There are certain tests all pregnant women have done by their obstetrician. Zinc and vitamin D are not considered standard of care yet. Thyroid function tests, or TSH, is standard of care and that's something that needs to be looked at. Again, I might be a little more picky about what I want to see in terms of good thyroid function. I am looking for TSH, or thyroid-stimulating hormone, to be between 1.5 and 3.0. We don't want women during pregnancy to be hypothyroid. Hypothyroidism during pregnancy and early childhood is the number one cause of mental retardation in the world.

DB: I had no idea about that.

AU: Yes, we need to make sure our thyroid is working well to develop our endocrine and neurological system in the right way. Many moms of children who develop autism have a condition called Hashimoto's thyroiditis, which is an autoimmune condition where the body fights its own thyroid and in turn causes symptoms of hypothyroidism or low thyroid. Hashimoto's is an autoimmune condition against the thyroid. This condition will also predispose you to having a child with immune issues. Many doctors in the integrative world feel that Hashimoto's is strongly associated with gluten intolerance. If you have a history of Hashimoto's in your family or if you have Hashimoto's during your pregnancy, I strongly recommend you talk to your own functional medicine doctor about possibly avoiding gluten.

DB: If a mother is suffering from a chronic condition such as allergies, fibromyalgia, or colitis, is this something she should really try to maybe see a holistic practitioner or nutritionist before going on to get pregnant, if it is a planned pregnancy?

AU: Yes, I agree with that statement. I do believe that if you have a history of autoimmunity or immune issues then you're going to be at higher risk of having a child with immune or autoimmune issues. If you want to try and prevent that in a holistic fashion, then seeing an integrative practitioner would be very important in addition to your obstetrician during your pregnancy. Then you can work on addressing those kinds of immune issues in an integrative way. We are talking about cleaning up your environment and diet, preventing things that are going to trigger your immune system and create more inflammation. The two most inflammatory foods would be dairy and gluten.

DB: Let's talk about metabolic pathways because I really appreciated some of the information that you gave on the autism intensive webinar. I think most people are not aware, even though we say autism is not genetic it isn't to say that people don't have certain genetic variations that make them more vulnerable to certain problems and autoimmune illness. Can you explain the importance of metabolic pathways to parents that aren't aware of them and how when they aren't working optimally they can contribute to autism? Scott Smith touched on this a little, but I want to dive in a little deeper.

AU: There have been numerous studies, hundreds of studies in children on the spectrum having a higher amount of oxidative stress. Oxidative stress is a fancy word to explain that cells in our body are aging at a more rapid rate. It is kind of like a rusting process that's happening in the cells. The cells are not performing the way they should be because there is too much oxidation and not enough antioxidants. Again, numerous studies to show metabolically that kids on the spectrum have severe oxidative stress, seventy percent of them have low glutathione, and glutathione is a protein in the body that is the number one antioxidant. Obviously if you are not making enough glutathione, your body is going to be more predisposed to oxidation and therefore more damage to your DNA, RNA, and other cells.

The other thing glutathione does in addition to being a really important antioxidant: it helps with detoxification in the body. That means that glutathione combines with various chemicals and metals and escorts them out of the body through the liver to be released outside of our system. The key to their production of glutathione is a process called methylation and sulfation.

It is a process that occurs in all the cells in our body. Research shows that children with autism do not have a properly functioning methylation system. They are finding genetic weaknesses in the methylation pathway. These genetic weaknesses in methylation that lead to low glutathione and oxidative stress are further burdened by a toxic burden in the mother and toxins in the environment of the child. This then causes more oxidative stress and more damage to our cells. In addition, toxins from the environment have difficulty leaving the body, which causes more oxidative stress which results in a vicious cycle.

DB: We have touched on some of the genetic anomalies such as the MTHFR. Could you explain the relevance of these mutations for people who might not understand?

AU: The term for these common genetic anomalies—and these are not genetic disorders—is single-nucleotide polymorphism or SNPs, S-N-P-S. These single-nucleotide polymorphisms are called polymorphisms because we all have them, they make us who we are. For instance, if you have a family history of immune issues you probably have genetic polymorphisms in genes for your immune system. If you have a family history of Alzheimer's, you probably have genetic polymorphisms in genes that affect Alzheimer's. If you have a child with autism you as a parent also may have genetic polymorphism in methylation and glutathione production.

These genetic polymorphisms or SNPs are in certain genes and these genes code for specific enzymes associated with methylation. One of the most important genes that we look at is a gene called MTHFR or methylenetetrahydrofolate reductase. Now the methylenetetrahydrofolate reductase gene, codes for the enzyme, methylenetetrahydrofolate reductase. This enzyme helps to make an active form of folate called methylfolate. If you have a single-nucleotide polymoprphism or a SNP in this gene, instead of the enzyme working one hundred percent that enzyme might work less than fifty percent or twenty-five percent. When we look at these genetic anomalies in MTHFR we are looking at two specific genes.

DB: What are these mutations specifically referred to and who do we get them from?

AU: One is the MTHFR C667T and the other is MTHFR A1298C. Now if the MTHFR 677 gene is weak that means you have a polymorphism from mom and a polymorphism from dad. The term for weakness on both sides is called homozygous, or a plus+/plus+. If you have a MTHFR plus/plus with a 677 mutation, then that enzyme is going to work at about twenty-five percent capacity instead of one-hundred percent. Your body is going to have a lot of difficulty making methyl-folate. And what they find from studies from the Mind Institute is that if moms carried that gene, MTHFR 677 plus/plus, they are six times more likely of having a child with autism, especially if they don't take their prenatal vitamins because they need that folate.

As I've mentioned MTHFR codes for a gene that makes an enzyme that helps make methylfolate. For those moms folate is extremely important, the type of folate is also extremely important because of that gene defect. If you just take plain folic acid it may not make it through that enzyme because it is only working at twenty-five percent. Instead of using regular folic acid, these moms may need to use an active form of folic acid like methylfolate.

DB: So if you test positive for this anomaly is there anything that you can do to make it work better?

AU: Yes, as we discussed the issue of aberrant methylation is common in children on the autism spectrum. The two genes that have been really looked at are MTHFR and another gene that we haven't talked about yet is MTR or MTRR, which is methionine synthase. Methionine synthase is a gene that's associated with developmental issues as well and ADD. Methionine synthase is a gene that is methyl B12 dependent. So this combination of problems with folate chemistry and the problems of methyl B12 go on to create issues with glutathione and oxidative stress.

DB: How can people get tested for that one?

AU: Parents can get tested for these SNPs, regular laboratories can test for MTHFR. There are some specialty labs like 23andMe that parents can get tested for other genes including MTR/MTRR. Doctor's Data also does SNPs testing and more and more laboratories are doing testing on these SNPs. If you know your status of these genes then you can bypass your predispositions with the proper nutrition and focus on targeted cofactors of these enzymes. You can use certain minerals or certain vitamins. For instance, if you have a MTHFR mutation to bypass that mutation, the supplement that could potentially help the most is methylfolate.

If you have a MTR or MTRR mutation, you could bypass that weakness with methylcobalamin or methyl B12 supplements. These two genes are really important to know in terms of your status, if you have a child on the spectrum and you are thinking of having more children. Again, I just want people to realize that you can't just look at one gene and say, "This is a problem, this is what is the cause, this is the treatment." These genes interplay with one another and these supplements interplay with one another. I think that it is important to educate yourself, but also not be naive and say, "Okay, well it is just these two genes that are playing the biggest role." They do play a big role and they do need to be addressed but all the other stuff needs to be addressed as well.

DB: I also wanted you to touch on another pathway that does not get talked about as often. Please let people know about the significance of the sulfation pathway?

AU: If you think about gears on a bicycle, what we have is the methylation pathway interfacing with another gear, which is this folate pathway, which we talked about with MTHFR. But right underneath the methylation pathway is your sulfation pathway. So when methylation turns like a gear or like a hand on a clock, it also feeds the sulfation pathway. The sulfation pathway starts with an amino acid called cysteine. Cysteine then goes on to make various sulfur compounds, it makes something called taurine, which is really important for our bile and our gallbladder to emulsify fat. Cysteine makes an amino acid called alpha-lipoic acid, which is another important antioxidant. It also helps with the detoxification of metals in our body.

Cysteine goes on to make glutathione. It's a rate limiting step for making glutathione, which is that very important antioxidant and detoxifying agent in our body. The other pathway that cysteine feeds is the pathway that you mentioned called sulfation. Basically then cysteine makes these groups called sulfate groups. Sulfate groups are important for getting rid of our hormones, they are very important for getting rid of compounds called phenolic compounds, which are found in foods and chemicals. So if that sulfation pathway is weak or depleted our body may have trouble getting rid of pesticides, herbicides, and handling certain foods that are high in phenols.

Sulfate also acts like Scotch tape. It helps cells stick together. If we don't have enough sulfate, you have leakiness. A leaky gut, or leaky lungs would cause asthma, leaky skin would cause eczema, and a potentially leaky blood brain barrier could have far worse results. We want things that should be in the brain to stay in the brain, and things that should be in the body to stay in the body.

A very simple tool that families can use to help that sulfation pathway is Epsom salt baths. Epsom salts are magnesium sulfate and we need that sulfate. When our kids are toxic, sometimes their systems and these enzymes get blocked. It seems like the system gets stuck at sulfite and never makes it to sulfate in the chemistry. We really need that sulfate.

DB: I loved the things that you mentioned about this pathway and how it can lead to other things like asthma. So for people who don't have a child on the spectrum already but are concerned and have different various things in your family from an epigenetic standpoint. What are some supplements that would be good for someone to speak to their pediatrician about for any child to take, not necessarily one that has a child on the spectrum already. It seems like there are certain ones that are just good for any child to prevent illness.

AU: Right, because we talk about genetics and epigenetics and the environment what were talking about that could potentially prevent autism, it could potentially prevent other chronic diseases. What we are talking about is just getting the body in balance, getting the immune system in balance, getting methylation in balance, getting the microbiome in balance. When you do that no matter what you have, it can help. Whether it is asthma, allergies, eczema, or arthritis.

When you have a chronic inflammatory condition, it is then these types of tools that we are talking about that can help any of those things. So whether it is bronchitis, dermatitis, colitis, arthritis, or some other inflammatory condition, I can't say this enough but you've got to clean up the environmental burden. You've got to look at your nutrition and your diet. We do not want to add more inflammation to that system with genetically modified foods, trans fat, oxidized fats, and fried foods. You really want to eat good fats, fresh fruits, and vegetables, nutritionally dense foods. You want to stay away from inflammatory foods like casein and gluten, sugar and simple carbohydrates. I think that working on cleaning up your environment and cleaning up your diet are the most important things to do.

Number three would be cleaning up the gut. I really believe the gut is the key to overall health. For me, the most important supplements for cleaning up the gut would be digestive enzymes, probiotics, fiber, and herbs to help keep the good bacteria and the bad bacteria in place. In my world there are other tools that we use, but in terms of kids, probiotics and digestive enzymes would be a good place to start.

Then it is important to get the detoxification pathways working better. By working on the methylation pathway with potentially methylating agents like dimethyglycine, methylfolate, or methyl B12. And supporting the sulfation pathway with nutrients like NAC (nacetylcysteine) or Epsom salt baths. I also like the form of glutathione called liposomal glutathione. Again, it just depends on the child, their illness, and your history, how far you go with these things. But the basics would be environment, diet, gut health, and some immune supportive agents like zinc, vitamin D, vitamin C, and omega-3.

DB: The other thing I want to talk about is the concept of ongoing maintenance for prevention. So take someone like my daughter for instance who had eczema and food allergies. I addressed them and she hasn't had eczema in three years. But I still do a lot of work in terms of prevention. I am always watching her, and I continue the supplements even though she no longer suffers from a chronic illness and has no symptoms. Can you explain a little bit about how we live in this toxic world and the importance of maintenance?

AU: I have a whole series of lectures that we give in our practice called "Raising a Healthy Child in a Toxic World." It is an ongoing process. As I mentioned I have four children, three of my children have severe immune and autoimmune conditions ranging from allergies, asthma, type 1 diabetes, arthritis, and multiple chemical sensitivites. I've been doing this for twenty-five years and I'm constantly in this process of figuring out how I can keep the environment clean for my own children. Not bringing toxic cleaning agents, soaps, shampoos, detergents into my home, even furniture, feeding them good quality water, good quality food—it's an ongoing process.

DB: I want to go back to one significant thing that is very common in this country and it happened to my son, which is jaundice at birth. Can you talk a little bit about why in some cases that might be something significant or an early warning sign. Nancy O'Hara touched on it but I would like to discuss it more in depth.

AU: When people use the word jaundice, what are we talking about? We are talking about bilirubin not leaving the body as quickly as it should. And that is a symptom of the liver not starting up as quick as it needs to or not doing what it needs to work efficiently. When we see that, our first thought should be: okay, is my child receiving an extra load of something that he or she can't get rid of and what can I do to keep that liver moving and flowing. If it is extremely severe then the pediatrician uses bili lights in the hospital to kind of help clear that excess bilirubin.

Adults and older children are less likely to become jaundice rather than a young baby, but they still might have a problem with the liver being a little stressed out. One of the symptoms we see with a stressed out liver is aggression or brain fog in some of our patients. If they have some of these symptoms, we tell them to do something called a castor oil pack. It is a really simple technique where you take a piece of cloth, you drizzle it with castor oil, you place that on top of the liver and then you top off that cloth with a little bag like a Ziploc bag, and then a heating pad for fifteen minutes. The heat draws the castor oil into the liver and gallbladder and essentially improves circulation to kind of flush out any back up in the liver and in the gallbladder.

Castor oil is high in an acid called undecylenic acid, which is anti-inflammatory and it is antimicrobial as well. That is a tool to help and I would think that would help a little jaundice baby too. I just haven't had enough experience to give to babies because now my practice I see mostly children on the spectrum. It is a very simple, easy to do, and no side effect type of tool.

DB: I know that you deal with a lot of children on the spectrum so I wanted to ask you if there are a lot of parents like me who are mindful of trying to prevent it in their next child. And what type of things do you ask them to do differently? Do you do any special testing or special supplements in hopes of preventing?

AU: We do have a lot of families in our practice and I get that question a lot from moms who want to have another child. We want moms to avoid exposure to a lot of toxins, chemicals, pesticides, even from makeup that may contain phthalates, BPA, and parabens. In addition to that environmental cleanup, we ask moms to clean up their diet. I urge them to be on dairy-free, gluten-free, organic diet with plenty of good fats and avoiding trans fats and oxidized or fried fats as well.

Women should continue to exercise if they have been exercising, getting the oxygen flowing to their bodies. And then trying to be stress free, which is very difficult when you have a child on the spectrum. Obviously you are going to be worried to death about what is going to happen to your other child, but be mindful, try to stay positive, do things for stress reduction. Whether it's prayer, singing, or yoga, whatever parents can do to de-stress during that very stressful time.

In terms of pregnancy, the big things for our patient population would be to make sure your microbiome is healthy. If you've got yeast overgrowth, addressing that, if you've got Group B beta strep, trying to address that naturally without antibiotics early on, eating fermented foods and cultured foods. Supplement-wise: taking your prenatal vitamins, supplementing zinc if necessary, and then taking an active form folate and an active form of B12. If you had a child on the spectrum, potentially folinic acid or methylfolate for folate and methylcobalamin for B12, in addition to what is in the prenatal vitamin. I would think those are the important supplements. Plus I'm a big fan of DHA for pregnant women, babies need DHA or omega-3 for proper brain development. Make sure you are getting about one gram or one thousand miligrams of omega-3s during your pregnancy.

DB: Then once the baby is born of course you hope that the mother can breastfeed and the baby can get all these wonderful nutritional supplements and nutrients from her diet through the breast milk. If she is not able to breastfeed or continue breastfeeding, do you check the child for certain levels and put the child on supplements?

AU: Yes, with women if they are nursing, the vitamin D that they are taking gets into the breast milk and then the child will get the vitamin D and omega-3 that way. Now, I think some of the baby formulas supplement with omega-3 and put it in the baby formulas. I think for the babies the main thing would be adequate amount of vitamin D. A safe amount of vitamin D to give a baby would be four hundred international units if we are concerned or potentially get a blood test.

Dr. Usman wrote a wonderful article about autism prevention in the *Autism File* Magazine with her coauthor Beth Hynes called "Avoiding Autism." One of the best things they included was a very user-friendly chart of pregnancy dos and don'ts. They have graciously given me permission to print it in my book. Please take a look at their many wonderful tips below:

DO	DON'T
Eat organic, hormone-free food	Consume fish or foods with MSG or food dyes
Drink organic green tea, filtered water, and antioxidant rich organic juices	Drink soda, carbonated beverages, or alcohol
Use stevia, raw organic honey, and xylitol as sweeteners	Consume artificial sweeteners
Go for walks and get some sunshine daily	Be exposed to lawn chemicals or secondhand smoke
Use aluminum-free natural deodorant in them	Use moisturizers or makeup with chemicals or parabens
Use natural hennas to color your hair	Use chemical dyes, perms, or other such hair treatments
Use cast iron, glass, or stainless steel cookware	Cook with pans that are non-stick, Teflon-coated, or made from aluminum
Use chemical-free cleaning products in your home	

DO	DON'T
Yoga and engage in stress management techniques, such as massages and listening to soothing music	Start a rigorous exercise program, sit in a sauna, or get dental work (not even cleanings)
Eat fermented foods, cook with organic coconut oil, use organic raw apple cider as salad dressing, and consume healthy fats and cold-pressed oil	Wait until labor arrives to discuss NOT subjecting your baby to vaccines
Use natural remedies for pain, like homeopathic arnica	Talk on a cell phone without a headset or work with a laptop computer on your lap
Drink kombucha and take probiotics	Undertake a major home renovation (concern is for lead and other toxins in the process)
Run an air filter in your bedroom while you sleep	

DO	DON'T
Invest in an organic baby mattress, bedding and pillows, and hypoallergenic encasements	Clothe the baby in pajamas soaked in flame-retardant chemicals
Bathe your baby daily in warm filtered water—enjoy the experience with your baby!	Use soaps, moisturizers, or other "baby products" on the skin as such items are unnecessary and contain harmful chemicals
Feed with all organic and hormone-free products	Introduce dairy, gluten, or soy until after age two
Feed baby using glass bottles	Feed baby from plastic bottles or cups, or microwave formula or breast milk
Wearing a hat, walk outside with baby to get ten to fifteen minutes of sunshine daily	Take your infant into polluted and heavily populated locations
Run an air filter in baby's bedroom	

I remember first hearing about these genetic variations and the metabolic pathways they influence, during my son's initial visit with Dr. Nancy O'Hara ten years ago. These SNPs have been very well known and studied in the autism community for quite some time. It's interesting that mainstream doctors will check for them in certain instances; however, most of them do not know what type of recommendations to make once they find out that you are positive for one or two copies. The good news is that they are familiar with the test and will most likely have no problem ordering the lab work to check for it. However, you will still need to speak with someone knowledgeable that can tailor an individual plan just for you, especially if you are already pregnant. Remember, it's best to work with a nutritionist or functional medicine practitioner that has a lot of experience with autism and other chronic health issues, so they will know exactly how to advise you with similar recommendations like the ones given by the practitioners in this book.

Please keep in mind that even if you are positive for these genetic SNPs, it is not the end of the world nor does it mean that your baby will definitely develop autism or some other chronic illness. It merely gives you information that you should try to support these pathways to make them work better in order to give your baby the best chance of preventing autism. Information is key and using it to your advantage will help tip the odds in your favor, and that's all you can ask for. My hope is that in describing that your genes are not absolutely sketched in stone, you will feel empowered that you have some control over whether or not you develop an illness. Please believe that your choices do matter and they can influence your body to stay in balance or get out of balance. Disease cannot flourish when the body is in homeostasis. So look for the little signs that Dr. Usman talked about as far as digestive upset, allergies, or eczema. When these "symptoms" are displayed, your body is trying to get your attention. It is saying, "Hey take a look at me, the immune system is off kilter and needs to be put back on track."

I look back at my daughter and she had so many of these soft signs in the first couple years of her life. And this occurred with me doing so many preventative measures such as homemade baby formula, specialized testing and supplementing with probiotics, fish oil, and vitamin D, etc. I know in my heart, had I not been so vigilant that she may easily have gone down the same path as my son. She had so many of the contributing factors, but I stayed focused on the ones that I could help and control. Even with all the recognition and testing that we did, it was still such an intense fight like we were sinking in quicksand. I am grateful to all the practitioners who helped pull us out and saved her.

To this day, I explain to her all the time how her brother saved her. Sometimes I feel that she isn't being sensitive to him when he is having a particularly tough time and I use that moment to remind her how lucky she is that we learned so much from our experience with Dylan. This is the reason I am writing this book so we can continue his legacy. My son has helped so many children to not suffer the same fate as he has. It is important to me that he does not suffer in vain.

I don't expect that you will be able to do every little thing that we have mentioned and please don't beat yourself up for the things you can't. By the fact that you have picked up this book, I know that you are already way ahead of the game. You are a conscious thinker, one that wants the very best for your child, and someone that will go out of their way to do things that are not necessarily convenient or conventional. For this, your child is very lucky.

As a conscious thinker, you recognize the importance of individualizing treatment. And making individual choices about the health of our children is exactly why the next chapter was so vital for me to include on vaccines. I take a deep breath as I write this, since the very thought of the subject seems to conjure up so much angst in people. I only want the best for all of you and your families. For this reason, it is so important that I give you the information that some of you won't have heard anywhere else. You should take in the information and make your own decision, just as you will for every other aspect that we have spoken about in this book. You will decide what to eat, which personal care products and cleaning supplies to purchase, where you will live, and whether or not you will follow the CDC-recommended vaccination schedule. Your life is governed by the choices **YOU** get to make. Remember that your opinion is the most important one to listen to.

CHAPTER SUMMARY

Cleaning up your diet is one of the most important steps to preventing illness and protecting your health. Moms should consume organic food, healthy fats, and lots of fruits and vegetables especially during pregnancy.

It is extremely important to stay away from GMOs and pesticides.

It is a good idea to supplement with probiotics, fish oil, and vitamin D.

Mothers with autoimmune issues should consult with a functional medicine doctor to deal with those immune issues.

Your genes don't determine whether or not you will get a chronic illness. They interplay with the environment, which is the study of **epigenetics.**

Listen to your intuition and don't second-guess yourself when it comes to your children, even if the pediatrician says, "Don't worry everything is fine."

Look for the signs that the immune system is imbalanced since there is so much you can do to fix it before the damage goes deep.

You can check for SNPs and do things to make your methylation and sulfation pathways work better, such as B12 and methylfolate.

Consider having your copper-zinc ratio tested.

Try to reduce stress, especially during pregnancy.

Chapter 10

WHAT YOU MIGHT NOT KNOW ABOUT VACCINES
with Jack Lyons-Weiler, PhD

There is absolutely no way that I could get through writing a book on preventing autism and not bring up the subject of vaccines. It's almost as if the two are synonymous these days. Vaccines seem to conjure up some of the most intense feelings in people no matter what side you are on, and for that reason I don't want to spend too much time on my own opinion. The point of this chapter is to give you information and data that is not readily disclosed to the public. However I do want to mention that I did suffer a vaccine reaction in 1999 when I was thirty years old, and my son had multiple vaccine injuries culminating with the one that left his brain damaged by a stroke in 2005, catapulting him into the abyss of autism almost instantly.

In my personal experience, I went to Lenox Hill Hospital during the summer of 1999 in the middle of the night to have a plastic surgeon give me two stitches to sew up a tiny cut above my right eye lid which in his words was, "one that did not need any stitches at all." I admit to being very vain at the time and insisting on stitches from a plastic surgeon to make sure my face was camera ready for my job as an on-air television news reporter. Somehow in the course of this visit he decided that I needed a tetanus shot for this cut that "did not even require stitches." The logic behind this did not make any sense to me, but I was more preoccupied with not having a scar on my face. So I allowed him to administer the vaccine, since back then my former self did not question any doctor's treatment plan. At the time, I remember my biggest fear was that my arm would be sore and it might be difficult to hold the camera or mic over the next few days, since I vaguely remember this type of intense soreness happening to me as a child. Never did I imagine that shot would alter the path my life took forever.

Almost immediately I noticed that I became itchy whenever I was outside in the sun. Next it seemed that every smell within 50 feet seemed to bother me, from people's perfume right down to the ink on a newspaper that someone sitting a few seats away on a bus might be reading. Over time it became increasingly difficult to ignore how much my life was changing. I refused to go to the movies or theater where I would be around a lot of people, and quite frankly I even developed a persistent fear that I might get trapped in an elevator with someone who had just doused themselves with too much cologne. It may sound funny on paper, but there was nothing humorous about how debilitating my life had become. Most doctors that I went to during this period of time felt that it was all in my head, so I just gave up going to them. What was the point? I knew it was real and they just made me feel awful! Well as bad as this vaccine reaction seems, it was nothing compared to what my baby boy experienced and still feels the effects of today.

As I mentioned in the beginning of the book, I was not able to get pregnant for the longest time and as you can see I was quite sick. Looking back now, I am amazed that IVF even worked for us on the first try. I was pretty reluctant and nervous about vaccines while I was pregnant with my son. People were just starting to connect them with autism and other health issues. I spent a lot of time during my pregnancy reading books about vaccines. I wanted to make a really informed decision just like when I read hundreds of reviews online and visited consumer reports to read up on the safest car seats. Somewhere deep inside of me, I had such an uneasy and bad feeling about giving vaccines to my baby. Every member of my family has had some sort of reaction to a pharmaceutical product at one time or another, so this made me especially nervous. I also never did well taking over-the-counter medication either. I think some people are just too sensitive to anything synthetic or chemical. My mother also died after taking a prescribed antidepressant. I watched in horror as she tried to kill herself every day for twenty-three days straight during that fateful summer in 1984. I was only thirteen years old and should never have seen what I saw that day. Now many years later, that same drug has a black box warning saying that it may increase suicidal thoughts and ideation. I have also read documents that the company knew many years before that this was a side effect of the drug. So you can see why I might not have had full trust in the same companies that were making vaccines that I was supposed to inject into my perfect little healthy baby.

I would never tell another person what medical decisions to make for their child. One of the most difficult things about being a parent is having to make all these decisions and hope that we had enough good information at the time on which to base them. I know you have heard countless times how wonderful and safe vaccines can be; unfortunately this isn't always true for everyone. And it was not true for my son Dylan. He suffered a stroke after his eighteen-month Hib shot. I will never ever forget that day.

I still remember the clothes that he wore that afternoon. A picture of what he looked like before his vaccine injury will be etched in my mind forever. It's important that you hear his story, even though thousands of children are vaccinated each day with no incidents at all. Because as parents we have to weigh the risks for everything our children do, since ultimately we will be responsible for every outcome and have to take care of them no matter what.

Here is Dylan's story: I took Dylan to his pediatrician's office for his eighteen-month well visit. I had been doing a very alternative vaccine schedule and was only giving him one shot at a time. He still had a bad reaction each time I let them administer any of them, which can be seen in his medical records. I would ultimately end up returning to the pediatrician a few days after each visit that he had received a vaccine. At one point, I had taken a pretty long break, maybe six months or so since his last one. I knew that I would be applying to nursery schools and felt intense pressure that I was so behind. At this point, he had only received six shots total, which wasn't even one full round that they give to babies. So I reluctantly made the decision that it was time to get going again. Dylan had already received one Hib shot previously, so I wasn't too worried about him having a really bad reaction. Well immediately after the nurse left the room, I sensed something wasn't right. He looked white as a ghost and very pasty. It was only a six-block walk home, but I must've stopped every half a block to walk in front of the stroller just to look at him. It was my mommy's intuition. Once we got home I fed him quickly, bathed him, and put him down to sleep. The next morning, something was really wrong and I never heard a sound out of him for the next seven years. Not only did he lose his speech, but his gross and fine motor skills also unraveled over the next couple weeks. He could no longer walk up stairs. His eye contact disintegrated into nothing. There was no reciprocity and I barely thought he could hear me anymore. Most people experience a more regressive form of autism where the child loses skills slowly over a period of months and it's hard to tell what may have caused or contributed to it. Mine was literally overnight as if someone flicked off the light switch—and poof he was gone!

Slowly over time, I stopped seeing him smile and wanting me to pick him up. It felt like we existed in two very separate worlds. Anyone that I mentioned his situation to made me feel like I was overreacting, including his pediatrician. If I could just go back and change the course of that one day. There are moments that I look at his baby pictures and think how the world was his oyster. I tear up as I write this. I know intellectually that it's not my fault, but I made the decision to bring him to the doctor. I walked into that room, held him tight and let the nurse inject him with that fateful shot. I changed the course of his life forever! To say that I feel a little guilt on some deep level would be such an understatement. I have no choice but to forgive myself everyday, which is probably why I work so tirelessly to try to recover him. I feel that if I can get him better maybe it will set me free again.

Please know that I don't tell you this story to scare you away from administering vaccines. Again we all have to make tough decisions as parents every day, and these are individual choices, so what is good for one child may not be right for another. I am not against anyone doing vaccinations. However they are not safe for my son and me. He has two MTHFR genetic variations that make his ability to detox the chemicals and adjuvants in them very difficult, and the same goes for me.

I realize that some of you may not want to hear this "downside of vaccines," so feel free to just skip over this chapter if you please. For those of you who would like to have both sides of the story, I have chosen an esteemed scientist who will present some of the facts that you may not have heard before. We are going to arm you with information, including links to some of this important information, so that you can do some more research on your own if you choose to.

Jack Lyons-Weiler is a well-trained scientist that kind of got into the subject of vaccines by accident. He explained to me in our interview that he had just written a glowing chapter all about how wonderful vaccines are when the story about the whistleblower came to light, which he will explain the details of and how it initiated his journey to question everything he thought about vaccines. He started for the first time to really look at the research and the science behind vaccines and had some new assertions and revelations about them. He is now working tirelessly to educate those in power how he feels that we need a return to objectivity in science on the question of vaccine safety, they can and should be made safer, which is something I am sure we all want. I can't imagine for a moment that any of you readers don't care that my innocent son was injured.

I would also like to disclose that Jack has two fully vaccinated children. Here is our interview:

DB: Are autism rates rising?

JLW: Autism rates are rising, yes. First of all, on first principles, there is no possible way that a genetic explanation of autism could increase in the classical sense of the heritability of risk of autism at the rate that we see the reported rate of autism increasing. A caveat there is that twenty percent of kids with ASD diagnosis have increased copy number variations. Second, research has shown that changes in diagnosis do not explain the full scope of the increase. Those changes happened a while back now, and the rates are still increasing.

DB: A lot of people have not heard about the situation concerning the vaccine whistleblower from the CDC. Can you tell us a little bit about William Thompson and what did he come forward with?

JLW: My understanding of Dr. Thompson is at the time of the research studies that are in question, he was a senior research scientist at the CDC, intimately connected with and engaged in firsthand involvement and responsibilities on association studies that focused on the question of whether or not either rates of autism were increased in vaccinated individuals versus unvaccinated, or were rates of vaccination in autistics increased relative to rates of vaccination retrospectively in neurotypical individuals. In the conduct of that research, he published papers, more than people know, he published a number of additional papers as well with his supervisor, Frank DeStefano, concluding and forwarding the idea that there was no association whatsoever between any type of vaccination and autism.

What I've come to know by researching various sources is that Dr. Thompson stepped forward, as I understand it, to Dr. Brian Hooker with concerns that Dr. Hooker was going to find association in data that were released to Dr. Hooker under the Freedom of Information Act. The data that were released to Dr. Hooker came, as Dr. Hooker relays it, after ten years of the request from Freedom of Information release for the various studies in question, and these studies were done in the 2000s. Upon receipt of the data, Dr. Thompson, outside of the auspices of his position at the CDC—in other words, after work—contacted Dr. Hooker and wanted to speak with him. And Dr. Hooker managed to record Dr. Thompson with some stunning revelations on Dr. Thompson's direct involvement and his supervisor's direct involvement in the omission of results from studies that went forward into publication with the conclusion that there was no association of vaccination and autism. The vaccines in question there were the MMR vaccine for one of the studies.

The omitted results included the finding that African-American males who had received their vaccines on-time (i.e., according to the CDC schedule) had a higher risk of autism compared to those who did not receive their vaccines on time. This resulted in a strong association between autism and vaccination. And the data analysis plan, the original protocol that the study was founded on, was changed mid-game to change the inclusion criteria to include then only individuals who had valid birth certificates, which I'm not sure whether they were changed for other subgroups or not, but other subgroup analyses were conducted. The team led by DeStefano also left out results from idiopathic, or what they call "isolated autism"–individuals whose autism had no other co-morbid conditions, that really could only be explained by vaccination. The rest of the subgroup analysis results were also included in the study, not excluded, both in the published study and in presentations that I found in my research that Dr. DeStefano was giving at the time at scientific meetings.

In science, if we have conducted a study, it's really beyond the pale to cherry-pick those results that you want to put in your study, especially on something as critical as an observed positive association. In stepping forward to Dr. Brian Hooker, I believe Dr. Thompson was under the understanding that, at some point in time the things he was saying to Dr. Hooker would come forward. Dr. Thompson pointed to the specific data files that Dr. Hooker would eventually find a strong association. He also pointed to the statistical routines that may have been used, and I believe he intended to, although I'm not sure that he actually did, send the actual commands for his statistical package to the same exact analyses that were conducted by the CDC. Nevertheless, Dr. Hooker went ahead and analyzed the data and found the strong association that Dr. Thompson predicted he would.

Dr. Thompson also revealed other studies conducted by the CDC or on behalf of the CDC with colleagues that initially found strong association between vaccines and autism, only then to be delayed for a period of up to four years before release of the results, and then only after they found a way to make the association go away. There's a smoking gun email that has been released, where, in my view, it's quite damning. The title of the email is, "It just won't go away," meaning that the association won't go away.

DB: What did they mean by it won't go away?

JLW: What "It just won't go away" really reveals is that there is a design on the result that was required before publication, which is not science. We invest heavily in research, both through the NIH (National Institutes of Health) and the CDC and biomedical research at other institutions as well, the NSF (National Science Foundation) and the FDA, and there are certain common standards of behavior, acceptable norms of behavior, when it comes to handling issues like this. Holding onto a result for a long period of time and analyzing it and over-analyzing it and repeatedly analyzing it until you get the result that you want is really beyond the pale; it's grounds for dismissal at universities. If someone were found to do this covertly and then hide it and then deny it and the data is right there showing us that, yes they did that from an NIH-funded grant proposal, then there would be allegations of fraud. Papers would be retracted from statements of concern. We have a culture and protocol in science by which we handle these things. There have been people that have done these things in the past, and they have been sanctioned.

Unfortunately, nothing has really come from Dr. Thompson's revelations, and they're more than just allegations. They're actually a confession. He confessed that he was directly involved, but I've been reading about it, studying it, for some time and looking at the things that he says and looking at the other things that have come out, made available in part by Representative William Posey, it's become apparent to me that Dr. Thompson was under a great deal of duress while conducting these analyses, that he tried to do due diligence and to raise the issue knowing that his supervisors would not hear it. My take on it is from what I've seen. He went over his supervisor's head—he broke the chain of command so to speak—to the then-director of the CDC, Julie Gerberding. In so doing, he did not find relief for his concerns. Instead, for some reason, Dr. Julie Gerberding saw fit to allow Dr. Thompson to be reprimanded and suspended from his position.

It's interesting because Dr. Thompson reveals to Dr. Hooker in the discussion that at some point in time, Dr. Thompson had something of a mental breakdown. In some discussions with people that were involved in revealing Brian Deer in particular of Dr. Andrew Wakefield's earlier research where he had found a putative association between vaccines and gastrointestinal issues in autistics, Dr. Thompson's mental well-being was brought into question. I came to Dr. Thompson's defense and said that it was really distasteful for that topic to be treated that way because any ethical person in his position would feel a great deal of stress and under duress. People want to keep their jobs; they don't want to be pressured to do the wrong thing. You know, it is quite apparent that Dr. Thompson tried to do the right thing.

What I have to say about it is that I'd really like to see Dr. Thompson be able to come forward safely again in public, and I think his story needs to be told broad and wide about this culture of corruption at the CDC that he revealed to Brian Hooker. Personally, it's sufficient grounds for me as a scientist to have grave concerns over all the publications from that team and publications from scientists who have published with members of that team. The types of studies that they used were retrospective studies. The retrospective studies themselves individually are weak science studies; they're not randomized prospective clinical trials that are needed, required by the FDA for approval of new drugs and new procedures in medicine. Instead, they're retrospective, which are very plastic, amenable to biases, and easy to manipulate.

In other studies conducted by or funded by CDC on the question, there is a great deal of what I call "analysis to result," and specifically they continued to analyze it until they could find that they could make the associations go away. When they couldn't make the associations go away, they simply omitted the results. It's under any definition of scientific fraud, misconduct.

DB: It's interesting because the public relies on the CDC and its studies to know that there's no link between vaccines and autism, and that's what they believe. What kind of implications does this have for people to be able to trust this organization, CDC?

JLW: Okay, so I've thought long and hard about the sequelae, and they're actually quite large in number, and they're devastating. Let me start with the one that's really going to hit people's heart. First of all, our society is divided in the discussion between families or coworkers, there's this chronic stress, people who know full well that their child, for instance, underwent some kind of neurological change after vaccination, and for some reason it seems to be okay in our society if someone believes that vaccines might cause autism or contribute to autism to feel that there's something wrong with that person, that they're somehow crazy. Of course, these people are already tackling life with vaccine-injured children. Even if one can't buy into or doesn't accept that the vaccines may have contributed to or directly caused autism, these people already have a significant variable in their life, let's say, that they're dealing with. Of course, they want to find relief.

For me, it's very sad that we have this kind of conversation that is repeated thousands of times over, hundreds of thousands of times over. People are castigated, they're bullied, they're called names and marginalized. That's very, very sad because in reality, these are the people that the rest of us, who don't have vaccine-injured family members, really should be reaching out to help. Vaccines are effective at reducing infectious disease. And because they're effective at reducing infectious disease, my analysis of the over three thousand papers, studies on autism tells me that there is a genetic minority of people who are at substantial risk of adverse events from vaccines. That means that all of these individuals that have suffered one type of adverse event or another, if we all enjoy protection from disease from infectious pathogens, we've done that to a large extent at the cost of their personal suffering. They should be heralded as heroes.

That is not to say that autism as a condition is necessarily something everyone who is autistic is suffering from. It's not to say that every family that has an autistic child is bearing an unbearable burden, but it is to say that I believe that our society owes these people a debt of gratitude. These individuals are, in my mind, a diverse genetic minority, more susceptible to toxins in vaccines than the rest of us. Any benefit we gain from the use of vaccines we owe to their suffering. We therefore owe it to vaccine-injured individuals to make it right. I'm glad to know that the Vaccine Court finds some kind of vaccine injuries worthy of compensation, and that's appropriate.

The consistent pattern within the Vaccine Court, however, to not find direct causal links between vaccines and autism, is wrong. This has cost thousands of families any kind of real relief. In the Omnibus Hearings, there were five thousand families who were denied after finding an indirect causality of vaccines in five cases of autism. There have now been eighty-three cases given awards, which involved a diagnosis of autism. The consequences of the court's decision to determine that vaccines cause encephalopathy, and that autism is a sequalae of encephalopathy, but that somehow that means that vaccines do not cause autism cannot be sustained by logic. This move has been devastating to individual families who would otherwise be better able to, let's say, afford some in-home care or babysitters or therapies and treatments, education, while working. They could better afford a cleaner lifestyle for themselves and their children. The cost is two-fold because parents have to stay home and take care of their autistic children. Some would say "get to take care of them," and I certainly agree with that, but the cost to individual families is immense in America, because we won't have the association recognized.

I believe these people are entitled to compensation, they're entitled to our respect, and they're entitled to our gratitude. The consequences go well beyond the families and the kind of ongoing negativity in society that exists to persist and perpetuating this myth that there's no link between vaccines and autism. It includes a massive delay in research. First of all, there are no incentives to make vaccines safer. No one's asking questions. Okay, if vaccines contribute causally to cause autism, how do we prevent them from causing autism? That means that there are more and more cases of autism that are likely to occur in certain individuals as a direct result of this misleading scientific conduct.

DB: Can you tell us why there's no incentive, because parents who are reading this book might not have a vaccine-injured children?

JLW: There's no incentive because they are not held accountable for vaccine injuries. The National Childhood Vaccine Injury Act of 1986 gave them one-hundred-percent immunity from legal liability for any vaccine injury. So science on vaccine safety is corrupted. In fact, I would say that true vaccine safety science does not exist in the US. Okay, so in order for science to go forward, science is based on a logical series of events. The first that we do is we look at background knowledge. What do we accept as background knowledge? If we accept, say, that vaccines can contribute to autism, then a natural consequence of that would be to say, "Okay, well, perhaps we could find some biomarkers to find which individuals." Because autism is rare, the background knowledge on autism is rare. Now it's over two percent in our nation, but it's rare, still, one to two percent.

Background knowledge is that vaccines do or do not cause autism. If vaccines do not cause autism, then there's no reason to be concerned for screening to identify which people might develop autism from the vaccines. There's no incentive to look at the genetic information of those individuals to see if they have specific mutations that might cause one type of vaccine or another to be particularly dangerous for them. There are a number of good mechanisms that might cause that. But due to denial of reality, there's just no reason to do it. It wipes the slate clean. There's nothing to do in terms of protecting people from damage and injuries from vaccines.

In reality, I believe on the question of vaccines, we could have our cake and eat it too fairly easily. There's no incentive on the part of vaccine manufacturers, not just because there's no financial incentive, but because nobody's pressuring them to say, "Hey, you know what, we need to make vaccines safer!" They continue with the same formulations that are decades old. There's very little competition from newer, safer means of immunization. It's medieval science really to put metals into concoctions and inject them into people's tissues.

What we have is a lack of incentive to know more. There's no reason to ask questions, it stops people from asking scientific questions and we know a lot less about immunology, as a result. We know a lot less about the genetics of environmental toxicology as a result. I mean aluminum's a neurotoxin. Mercury is a neurotoxin. There are other additives in vaccines that are neurotoxins. These neurotoxins are not just found in vaccines. What could we have learned over the past fifteen years if the CDC and others accepted and promoted the idea that the science was telling them that, "You know what, vaccines may cause autism in some people." Okay, so let's find out which people.

Instead, they're stuck with the population level, and we're stuck with kind of palliative . . . "Okay, even if it does cause autism, it's a low risk, and everybody in America is kind of unrealistic. You have to live in a society where there can never be zero risk." I don't believe that is true. I don't believe that that's the case here at all. We all know that there's risks in life, but the difference between, say, natural risks of something happening to you and vaccine risks is that vaccines are man-made. We have the ability to control what goes into the syringe, what goes into a needle and through the needle into the body. We have the ability to concoct formulations that don't have additives that are dangerous, but there's no incentive to do that because there's no harm according to the so-called science. They may be more expensive, but added cost at the time of immunization can save billions in terms of the cost of neurological disorders to society. Remember, we're at 1 in 68, and newborns may now be as high as 1 in 25.

The other kind of negative consequences are, of course, potentially widespread autoimmune diseases. There's something like an estimated 1 in 5 Americans have an autoimmune disorder, and they're increasing. You look at classrooms they're filled with kids with atopic dermatitis, allergies, and many other autoimmune disorders. Most classrooms have an autistic child now, the consequences have been absolutely devastating. Every child with severe autism requires intensive therapy—that takes in many cases one full-time person per child. That adult caregiver or therapist could be contributing in other ways to our society.

DB: What ultimately changed your view on vaccines?

JLW: Sure, so I had written a book on Ebola, and in writing that book on Ebola, I found some red flags over some of the information coming from the CDC, inaccuracies. Then Director Tom Frieden, for instance, testified to Congress that there are no mutations in the Ebola virus, and he was sure that there was never going to be any outbreak because there are no mutations. At the time that I was listening to his testimony, I was working on the analysis of 396 mutations that have been previously published in the literature a month or so before. Initially, I figured, "Whoa, his science team is really not doing him well to keep him updated. There's 396 mutations, and here he is telling Congress that there's no mutations." Then I was invited, because I'm a scientist, as part of the scientific community doing research on Ebola, to a White House conference call. On that White House conference call, we were told that they wanted us to be sure that we were accurate in what we told the American public about Ebola because as scientists, people respect our opinion. We were then invited to ask any questions.

The first question was from a scientist, and she asked, "What was the CDC thinking in going to western Africa loaded for bear with all the suits on and so on without bothering to take advantage of the investment that we've made in western Africa in sociological and anthropological research?" We had scientists on the ground there that know the society very well, and instead of scaring everybody and just showing up, why not talk to them about who the community leaders are and so on. There were a couple of other questions at the end, and then I asked a question, "What about these 396 mutations? What do we know about them? Do they change their ability to detect Ebola? Do they change the virulence of the virus?"

The question was answered by a CDC scientist named Stuart Nichol who said that this virus in western Africa was the same as the virus from Zaire in 1995, so it was 99.999 percent similar, which I knew was not true. It's more along the line of 96.3 percent similar, about that, and so there was some potential very real differences. That kind of tipped me off that something was woefully wrong with the CDC.

Then I wrote a second book that had a chapter on vaccines in it, and I was kind of naively going to write a chapter on vaccines about how great vaccines were at saving lives and just tell the rosy story about how wonderful vaccines were for society and what a great translational success they were. It is one chapter, I think out of seventeen or eighteen chapters on a wide variety of topics. I wrote the first half of the chapter, and the first half of the chapter told the good side of vaccines, which were easy to recognize, and the second half of the chapter, I was going to write about the Wakefield incident and basically kind of repeat the standard party line if you will about our scientific fraud, and it was investigated, and so on. Of course, as I dug into it . . . it's ironic because it's about the same time as the Ebola outbreak was happening, Bill Thompson came forward with his revelations.

I ran smack dab into the Thompson affair, and being an objective scientist, I looked at all the evidence. I looked up all of the papers, I read the papers, I looked at the way that they handled the data analysis. I instantly recognized fraud. I looked for other evidence, and I could easily confirm with my own eyes that what Bill Thompson was saying was consistent with a very serious problem with the studies reporting the science being done on vaccines by the CDC. While I could see it right away, it took a long time for me to accept it. I didn't want to accept it. I wanted to get out of my book project and just finish the book clean and not get involved in something that was basically so potentially controversial or devastating, but then again, you know, I wanted the truth to be known. I wanted families to know. Anybody who bought my book, I wanted to be fair to the reader. I wanted to be a fair broker of knowledge and information because I'm a lifelong educator.

In that book, I not only concluded the chapter with the evidence that I thought was most important, and revealing the problem that

Thompson was revealing to Hooker, but also there's an addendum to the book that lays out four major controversies surrounding vaccine science. Most of them involve whistleblowers, so it was quite an educational experience for me. That book is *Cures vs. Profits*, published by World Scientific.

DB: Now, let's talk more about the vaccine injury compensation program because I think the most important thing is for people to have all the information to make that very personal important parenting decision of whether or not to vaccinate or do a different schedule. Are there vaccine injuries? Please explain the vaccine injury compensation program.

JLW: The vaccine compensation program was established, under President Reagan, ostensibly to make available funds for individuals who filed a petition claiming that they had a vaccine injury. This was after vaccine manufacturers threatened to get out of the business of making vaccines. There are a number of vaccine injuries that people could seek compensation for: these appear in the NVCP's vaccine injury table. This ostensibly freed pharmaceutical companies from liability, so that they were compelled by governments to create vaccines by contract because of the positive effects in protecting the population from infectious diseases. These companies also backed off of that, off that threat of leaving us without vaccines. It's a multibillion dollar industry. I don't think they would have ended their participation. They bullied the US government into these contracts.

In order to buffer that cost to them in terms of the value of their stock if there's something wrong with the vaccine, etc., the liability was taken away, and this is the solution that our government put up for people who have claims on vaccine injuries. They publish a vaccine injury table; in that table are the vaccine injuries that are recognized by the vaccine injury compensation program. If it's not on the table, then there's the high task of demonstrating and proving that there's actually what you're calling a vaccine injury of a family or an individual, that was caused by a vaccine. The burden of proof falls on the family. Autism is not found in that table. Encephalopathy is, but what doctor is going to give their patients with autism a diagnosis of encephalopathy?

DB: How is that possible?

JLW: What they did instead for autism is they ran a series of legal trials where they took typical subtypes of autism. They're not scientific subtypes or representative of other factors, but the idea was to have a handful of studies that they could then use to apply to a broad segment of the population who were claiming vaccine injuries leading to autism.

What they did consistently was probably, you might call it a "word salad," they all but say for some of these cases that vaccines cause autism. What they say instead is the vaccine induced encephalopathy, or encephalitis, which are not really diagnoses. Encephalopathy, anything with the "pathy" at the end of it means you have some kind of disease in the brain. Or "itis," encephalitis means that you have some inflammation in the brain. It doesn't point to the etiology or the cause, and it's not a real diagnosis.

You go to the doctor, and you say to the doctor, "I have a stuffy nose." He says, "Oh, you have rhinitis," it's a synonym for "stuffy nose." You're not doing anything special there except for putting a name on what they are telling you.

The national vaccine injury compensation program then says in some of these cases for instance, it had been argued that there had been mitochondrial dysfunction, and that the mitochondrial dysfunction was some kind of precursor to, and then the vaccines must have come in and done something, but without the mitochondrial dysfunction, perhaps you wouldn't have had autism, which may have well been true, but we know now that mitochondrial dysfunction can also be caused by vaccines.

Many of us have many mutations that are potentially contributing factors to disease-like conditions, and until we run into the toxin in the environment that we're susceptible to, we really don't have any kind of disease. So the ultimate cause was the environment, not the genes. In never actually saying and finding directly autism, what the national vaccine injury compensation master special court then does is it leaves us with a conclusion that the court has only indirectly found that autism can be caused by vaccines, which is a very narrow thin slice of logic, which I think is not sustainable over time. I mean, the more people push for mandatory vaccines and the more the political programs are out to put in mandatory vaccines, unless they change the vaccine formulas, then there's going to be more and more cases of vaccine injury. More and more cases of vaccine injury then are going to result in a stronger push for either compensation or better science of a true understanding of what's going on. Or both.

I don't think that the omnibus case decisions can really stand the test of time. To say that, "Yes, I drove my car through a red light, and it was a car accident. The bumper of a car went through the door, and it was the bumper of the car that hurt somebody; it really wasn't me. It wasn't my fault because the bumper of the car did it." You're bringing in these process descriptions to say that I only indirectly caused it because I'm not the one who caused the injury to that individual, it was my car, just doesn't wash in any other line of legal theory. I expect it all to be revisited some time.

DB: Is vaccine injury under-reported and is it affecting both children and adults?

JLW: I've looked at this problem for about a year now. Looking at it both as a citizen and talking with my fellow citizens and what the doctors tend to do when a parent goes to a doctor and says, "Listen, you know, my kid came down with this condition," and the doctors quite often give push back on, "Well, it probably wasn't the vaccine." Parents trust doctors. We entrust doctors with our lives. We pay them well, we have a good deal of respect for them given their training and their expertise, but we also have this feeling that we're putting our lives in their hands, and so we're trusting this person.

I have a great deal of respect for my colleagues and anyone in the medical community, but there is a lot of pressure to not attribute vaccine injuries through the vaccine adverse events reporting system. I've seen estimates that are as low as perhaps one percent of the number of vaccine injuries that occur actually make it into the passive reporting system. Most likely no more than ten percent of vaccine injuries are reported. What people don't realize is that you don't have to go to your doctor; anyone can file, use the adverse event reporting system. You just have to follow the instructions and be very careful, there are penalties if you falsely represent a vaccine injury in the VAERS. I think anybody that has a child that has undergone vaccine injury should consider not necessarily requiring the doctor's agreement. Just get your medical records, put a demand on the doctor's office for your medical records, don't mention vaccines per se, and then go ahead and make your report to VAERS. But we really need mandatory active reporting of all adverse events.

There are many kinds of vaccine injuries beyond autism, there's problems with neurological disorders, as I mentioned, encephalopathy or encephalitis is recognized, on the table. There's chronic arthritis, there's anaphylactic shock. You can get some kinds of infections from some vaccines that are directly related to the virus, like polio, that's recognized. People have gone into shock, and there are deaths. The risk is very, very small; I have to say that. The risk is small for death. It's very small, but it depends on the vaccine, and it depends on a lot of other conditions, not the least of which is genetic risk. While overall the risk of vaccine injury is not small and the risk of any one type of vaccine injury might be small, the risk for medium to serious adverse events considering all vaccines is however much larger. And when it happens to an individual, and it could be prevented, the risk is unacceptable. And the risk may be one hundred percent for some children. We need to find them, and protect them from harm.

There are also vaccine injuries that I believe should be on the table that are not yet on the table because the science doesn't really go forward that well. I mean, there's no national push to categorize and study all possible health outcomes that might be associated with vaccines. Instead, it's presupposed that rare vaccine injuries are just accidents and that because they're rare and that they might be easily confused with real adverse events. The attitude is "It might happen, but it's difficult to know, and so let's not study it." It's terrible, but they don't have the background knowledge correct. And the studies are not designed properly. If they grouped individuals with mutation in key genes together, and looked at rates of vaccine injuries, I expect the finding would be profoundly eye-opening. The science has to progress by asking questions, and we can't progress if we can't ask the question.

DB: Is this vaccine injury compensation program well publicized?

JLW: No, I didn't know about it. I don't think it's well publicized at all. I didn't know about it until I had to do some digging. I mean, people who have autistic children know about it, but the general population doesn't really know about it.

DB: Yes, unfortunately a lot of people find out about it after the three-year filing window has closed. Now I want to talk to you about safety testing of vaccines because a lot of people out there assume this rigorous testing has happened by the CDC.

JLW: Yes it's a shame. And doctors are trained that unless the adverse event shows up within twenty-four hours of vaccination, the changes in a person's health cannot be from vaccine. That's nonsense. First of all, when the CDC makes a statement on their website that vaccines do not cause autism, they're really relying on the MMR research. Not every individual vaccine has been tested for a relationship with autism. Not every childhood vaccine has been tested for being related to or not related to or associated with or casual of autism. Right there, we have a knowledge claim that's not founded on science to say it's not related to autism.

DB: Has the entire vaccination schedule ever been tested the way it is laid out?

JLW: No, there has not been a randomized clinical trial that says, "Okay, we're going to take one thousand patients that got this particular pediatric schedule and take one thousand patients that didn't get the schedule and see what the health outcomes are." These are important studies that need to be done.

         They have to be done with more than one thousand patients, though, because the risk is made small in part because there are genetic variants that might make some components of vaccines particularly toxic for some individuals. Some of them are very rare in the population, and so you have to have very large sample sizes to detect one percent, two percent adverse event. Because they rely on post-marketing surveillance for vaccine safety trials, they should be conducted looking at all health outcomes, not just the ones that we suspect.

DB: Have studies been performed to make sure that giving pregnant women vaccines is safe?

JLW: Then with respect to pregnant women, yes, there have been some studies. There have been some studies on some vaccines, likely there is acellular pertussis containing vaccine has been studied in pregnant women, but the sample sizes tend to be small, number one, and number two, they have exclusionary criteria. When they do these studies, quite often they'll exclude criteria that might predispose individuals to having an adverse event. In science, we do a study on a population, we're supposed to restrict our inferences about that study to the population that we studied. Let's say I did a study of, I don't know, hepatitis B vaccination on a Native American population. If I find that there is some kind of adverse event, then I'm not going to then say, "Okay, it applies to the rest of the world." I'll be concerned that it applies to the rest of the world, but I'm supposed to restrict it to that particular population. Well, here we have exclusionary criteria on these trials, and they turn around, and they make the inferences it's a global sweeping inference; it applies to everyone. It's just incorrect scientific logic.

Then the other thing is on the studies of pregnant women, they look at antibodies. They look at whether or not there are adverse events on the mother, but really haven't seen a lot of studies that show whether or not there are any adverse events in the fetus or in the baby. Quite often, there are high rates of spontaneous abortion after being vaccinated during pregnancy that are just kind of reported in the paper and not thought to be a big deal. Those are a big deal. If you're a family trying to have a baby, and you've got a fertility problem and you spend $22,000 and plus the emotional toll of losing a pregnancy, it's devastating. No, the science is nowhere near where it needs to be. We really, really need to move it up a notch.

The saddest part of all is that it's doable. We're told by the CDC, "Well, it's not practical, or we don't have the money for it." That's not how these government agencies should work. If they need the money for it, they should come to the people, and they should ask for it. There's no reason whatsoever why such studies couldn't go forward except that they probably suspect that there's going to be some verification of adverse events, and in finding these adverse events, then people are going to be scared and not get vaccinated. Then we'll have resurgence of infectious diseases. Nobody wants infectious diseases. They tend to make people sick, and people can die, and so then we should demand safer vaccines. It does no good to sweep the problem under the rug because this uncontrolled experiment that we're all involved in, and we're unwitting, unconsented into an experimental trial on these untested treatments.

The adverse events are now showing themselves, it's just a matter of time. I really do believe it's a matter of time, most Americans are going to know full well that vaccines can induce autism and many other types of adverse events. Unfortunately this knowledge will come at the expense of millions of affected individuals. But when it becomes obvious, free market forces should force the development of safer vaccines. Why not compete for market share on the basis of how safe newer methods of immunization might be?

DB: If someone wanted to get more information on vaccines to make a well-informed decision and look at some of the science that's out there, roughly how many peer-reviewed articles do you think can be found on PubMed that link chronic illness or autism to vaccines?

JLW: Okay, so we have to separate these into different categories. CDC doesn't really pay attention to animal studies, and yet they have no right to ignore animal studies. The FDA requires animal studies for treatments, of a new drug, for cancer. If there's an adverse event or toxicity of a drug in animal studies, in cancer, for say a new chemotherapeutic agent, the study doesn't go forward. That compound can't be brought forward, and the FDA wants to know the mechanism of action and of harm.

For the CDC simply to say, "Well, those are animal studies," or for anybody to say, "Those are animal studies, and animals are not humans, and they're different," they're technically correct that there are differences between animals and humans, and yet animals have the mammalian neurological system. Model animals such as mice also have the mammalian immunological system, and there are a great number of studies. I would say there are at least 150 to 200 studies that can be found, and maybe many, many more. Some of them are animal studies, and some of them are human studies. They not only show association, but some of the studies that I review in my book, among the one thousand or so studies that I cite in my book, tell us exactly how components like aluminum and mercury should cause neurological problems in mammals, and humans are mammals and therefore it should apply to us. With the animal studies and with the human studies that are available, there is plenty.

DB: A lot of people refer to a revolving door between the CDC and pharmaceutical companies. Have you heard anything about this to be true?

JLW: Well, I mean, Julie Gerberding, the former director of the CDC is now working for Merck. In terms of conflicts of interest, I'll just say this. I don't believe that anyone involved in vaccine research should own stock in any company that develops vaccines. They certainly should not be involved in the decision-making processes that bring vaccines onto a pediatric schedule while they own stock in a vaccine for a pathogen that's being considered for the schedule, or co-own stock or have a brother or sister that owns stock. These are things that are definitely happening in our country, and they absolutely should not happen. They should not be tolerated.

DB: What can be done about this?

JLW: People working in vaccine science, if you will, should pay attention to how the rest of the science is done. The rest of biomedical research requires that we recuse ourselves from certain situations. We can't review our own grant proposals. We can't review a grant proposal with people from our own institution. We can't review papers from people from our own institution or people that we've worked with in the past five years. We're trained. We train people in medical research how to handle these conflicts of interest. Conflicts of interest certainly can occur, they can occur by accident. I was working at one institution with somebody and we collaborated, and then they moved to another one, and then I'm on a grant review panel at the NIH, and I review their grant, and, "Oh, wait a minute. We're at the same institution. I worked with them. They're one of my recent collaborators. I can't do that." It's remarkably simple to recuse yourself from a situation. Nobody judges you for it. Nobody looks at you funny for doing it.

DB: Right now, in this country, a lot of states are trying to take away the religious exemption, they're trying to pass mandatory vaccinations for children. They have a plan to vaccinate all adults by 2020. We're finding that a lot of states where they're doing this, that the senators who sponsor it have been given large contributions by pharmaceutical companies. Is that something you're aware of?

JLW: I don't know of anyone, perhaps Senator Posey, who doesn't get contributions from pharmaceutical companies. That's part of the problem. You're going to find this kind of thing. I believe that the so-called anti-vaccine movement needs to be redefined. It needs to be redefined entirely into the Vaccine Risk Aware movement. Now, that doesn't mean that we're expecting all vaccines to be safe for everyone all the time, but what it means is that the individuals who are part of that movement are either anti-vaccine, which is their right, or they are one hundred percent behind vaccine safety. This is the vaccine risk aware community, and they are growing daily by the thousands.

If we don't get ahead of this and start demanding properly conducted vaccine safety trials, prospective randomized clinical trials, then the machine will roll over us, and we will see a sea, an ocean, of vaccine injuries that put a potentially fatal drag on society. I'm not just talking about autism. I'm talking lost work, lost productivity, lost wages, lost consumption, and certainly mortality and morbidity associated with it.

This is the decay of our society, and mind you, it's a moral decay. Anybody who wants to argue that it's not right to demand safer vaccine trials, well, if you say that you're one-hundred-percent pro-vaccine safety, what does that make any detractor? Are they against vaccine safety? If you're Vaccine Risk Aware, what does that make your critics? Or, do they think that me, a classically trained, rigorously trained scientist who spent my career advocating for objectivity in science just all of a sudden I've gone crazy? I've lost my mind?

These pejorative personal attacks have no effect on me. If somebody attacks me that way, they really don't know who they're dealing with. I'm not concerned about it whatsoever. There's many, many people who are concerned. They're afraid of losing their job. They're afraid of their coworkers losing respect for them. They're afraid of coming across like they're somehow crazy. In the meantime, there's money hand over fists, there's profits being made hand over fist. Something like $144 million a day is the last estimate that I saw in terms of profit from the vaccine industry, which I believe if the vaccines are safe and they were protecting us all from infectious diseases and making sure that they weren't harming a significant minority of people, they would be more than entitled to it.

DB: Now, you have written a book on the environmental and genetic causes of autism, and your book was recently published. Is there anything that you can tell us about those causes?

JLW: You commonly hear people saying that no one knows what causes autism. This is patently false. We know what causes autism. We know a plethora of things that can cause autism. There's a drug that is used to modulate depression, valproic acid, or valproate. When used gestationally, it causes autism. Thalidomide, when used gestationally, it causes autism. You don't hear about this. Why don't we hear about this? We don't hear about it because if you look at the mechanisms by which these drugs cause autism, and then you look at the mechanisms of what happens to the brain during development of mice or responses in brains that are measured in humans, when you have, mercury intoxication or if you have aluminum intoxication, it's the exact same mechanisms.

This is what I mean by saying that there are hundreds of studies that not only go beyond showing association; they show the mechanism, which is an order of magnitude higher in terms of level of evidence for the FDA. If you have a new drug for cancer and you think that it works, you have to show the FDA how it works. You can't just show them that, "Look, we have higher survivorship." They want to know the mechanisms.

In the book, I propose a theory; it's called the environmental toxin liability sampling theory. In this theory, it ties together all of the evidence from hundreds of studies of genetics of autism as well as environmental causes of autism. First of all, I can say autism is not a classically genetic disease. It is extremely rare that you're going to find an autistic parent that's given birth to or fathered an autistic child. There are certain traits that run in families. The risk of autism certainly has a high heritability itself, but it's not predominantly a genetic disease. There's no single autism gene or two or three autism genes. Second, of the hundreds of genes that appear to be related to autism in some way, there's really only a handful, and therefore a tiny percentage of cases of autism where we can say that the genes themselves contributed significantly to the risk of "genetic" autism.

Instead, what we see are many of the genes are environmental toxin susceptibility genes. They can't act alone in inducing autism in the absence of some environmental factor, or they're not likely to act alone. There certainly are some, like synaptic genes if you have two or three or four mutations in these kinds of genes, if you happen to be born with those mutations, then you're likely to get truly genetic autism. But that would be very, very rare.

The vast majority of the genes that contribute to the phenotype that we call autism or ASD modulate or change characteristics in people in the normal population as well, and so the three categories of genes are the true autism risk genes, and then you have the environmental susceptibility genes, and then you have genes that just control traits like intellectual ability or contribute to variation in intellectual ability. They contribute into that variation in the normal population, that is, the neurotypical population, as well as in autistic population. There are certain phenotypes, there are certain characteristics, of autistics that appear to be exaggerated, and they're just kind of exaggerated normal, if you will. The exaggerated normal characteristics aren't really autistic characteristics. What you have is an autistic brain, an autistic child, expressing normal population-based variation that comes out looking different because it's expressed in a different type of person. They're still human, they're still lovable. But the biology of their brains are distinctly different.

I look at the symptoms and diagnosis of autism, and I look at DSM-5 from the perspective of the geneticist, not as a psychologist and psychiatrist, but as a medical researcher. What I see there is a very odd administrative kind of erasure of regressive autism. I put the task to myself to find regressive autism in DSM-5, and it's there, it's in all the caveats. It's in the ifs, ands, and buts. Regressive autism, as you may know, is the most rapidly increasing type of autism, as opposed to natal autism, or congenital autism if you will. But no one is ever given a diagnosis of "Regressive autism" due to the administrative structuring of diagnosis.

I review in the book all of the evidence that I could find that shows that there's a genetic or epigenetic component to autism, and there's a great deal of that, but only about fifty percent of the variation in the risk of autism can be contributed to any kind of genetics or epigenetics, something that is slightly heritable. There are hundreds of, hundreds and hundreds of autism genes so to speak; the brain is very complex, and the immune system is incredibly complex. As I teach in my classes, there are many ways to break a gene. There are many ways to break a biological pathway. Then I go into which genes might be related to speech, language, and communication, phenotypes. I look at genetic and environmental factors influencing the social and cognitive skills.

I look at cognitive phenotypes. I look at the genes that might be contributing to repetitive motor behaviors and seizure phenotypes, those that are contributing to sensory phenotypes and immunological factors, and gastrointestinal, renal phenotypes for the kidney problems. One of the major findings that I have in the book is the gut-mind link. People are looking for some way that the gut might be influencing autism in the mind or the mind might be influencing the gut, less frequently, but there's certain cells in the brain that become activated, they're called microglial cells, activated by toxins, like aluminum and mercury, and other things like valproic acid, and Thalidomide, and so on. These then turn into little brain cell-eating machines, they chew away at the dendrites on the axons, and they kill neural precursor cells. They do brain damage, it's self-induced brain damage, but it's not like an autoimmune disorder of the classic type. This is an innate immunity, which means they have a series of chemicals that exist that are supposed to signal the macrophagic microglial cells to work in the brain. This is a form of innate autoimmunity, and it is preventable and reversible.

These microglial cells are not only active in the brain, but they're also highly active in the intestine. The same kind of cellular damage that we see in the nervous system and the brain we see in the intestines. This probably explains part of the link between the mind and the gastrointestinal changes. When a child has a leaky gut, they not only have loose tight junctions: they can have serious, chronic, and widespread intestinal lesion, and the barrier between the food environment and the bloodstream can be lost.

I review all of the evidence that shows mercury and autism, induced neurological damage in autism. I review all the vaccine studies and the autism studies that are ignored by the CDC. Then I go into some more conceptual mode, how to think about comorbidity. You know, people with autism are more likely to have certain kinds of subtypes of diseases, and how we think of that actually feeds back and influences how we do our science. In terms of defining effective study design going forward to understand autism, we really have to look at it from a phenotype perspective, not from a DSM-5 diagnostic perspective.

I've given a chapter on how logical it is to think about autism as a preventable condition and certainly as a treatable condition. You know, there's a division within the autistic community right now. There's some name-calling going on over whether or not autism is something that we should just accept and respect and not worry about treatment. No, I think we should accept and respect people, and there are people that get upset if you say you're going to cure autism. For them, it's not a treatable condition and that they're proud to be who they are. Well, they're entitled to that, to be proud of who they are, but I think that some of the treatments that are going to come out in the near future will allow them to be more of who they are, and that's a different view on that.

I outline a great number of ways to shut down those microglial cells, a large number of drugs, a large number of foods. Of course, none of it's medical advice. It's all done under the auspices of a review of the research. I close out the book with a call for better research in autism, from the perspective of causes. We really need to understand this. It's taking over a large segment of our society, and for us to continue to function as a compassionate and caring society, we certainly can't allow brain damage to continue unabated in the name of protecting us from infectious diseases, and I'm sorry if I offend anyone by saying the word "brain damage," but that's exactly what it is. We've got microglial cells that go and strip away dendrites so that they're single point-to-point synapses, instead of more complex synaptic architectures with multiple points. Those connections that are made during learning, instead of having multiple connections between brain cells, most of the brain cells in autistics are connected singularly, I mean, in severe autism. These differences have a profound impact on sensory experiences and cognitive functions.

DB: Yeah, just so you know, personally to add one more person to your list, I have no problem with you saying brain damage because that's what it is. Hopefully, in a lot of cases, it can be reversed, or at least some of it, and certainly in my son's case, it has been reversed, and I'm very happy about that. I guess the takeaway message from the book itself is going to be, for me, I want people to understand not to wait till it's completely broken to try to fix something.

JLW: Well, I review the most biologically significant genes that I could find that were studied. I think it's a great idea for anybody who has an autistic child in their family to have the child tested. It's good to know what you're dealing with, right? Are you dealing with a mutation that involves a synaptic gene? A mutation that involves a glutamate transporter? A mutation that involves mitochondrial dysfunction?

Intolerance of a specific environmental factor? You know, the rest of medicine is racing towards individualized medicine. I think a genome scan of known variations associated with autism is great. You know, even if it just allows you to know, "Wait a minute here, there was something genetic," it doesn't mean that the disease itself is genetic, and it doesn't absolve any environmental toxins. It may be incredibly important for children who have these scans, then, to also reach out into the research community and find medical researchers like myself who want to then try to study the genetic variations further with respect to which treatments work and which don't work. The more information you have, the better. There are companies out there that have panels you can order for autism risk. I don't think the panels are by any means comprehensive, and more are being added all the time. If I had an autistic child, I would have their entire genome sequenced and then any mutation that I thought was potentially interesting given what I know about genetics and autism, I would then have validated with a more clinical test.

The other point about the book, if we go back one question, is in the environmental toxin liability sampling theory. We're creating an environment where everywhere we turn there are more and more toxins for people to run into. I believe that the increase in autism that's occurring is simply because we're putting more and more toxins into our environment, more and more toxins into the vaccines, increasing the dose, vaccinating everyone, regardless of birth weight, using many vaccines at once, and we're just finding people who happen to be super susceptible to that kind of toxin in their environment. The susceptibility is genetic, but the disease itself is caused by the toxin. Many people who are thinking about genetics of autism want that to be the reverse. They want to say, "Okay, well, the genes caused it, and therefore it wasn't the toxin," but that's not how it really works. They think of the genes as the cause, and the toxins as trigger. But if you work out the logic, they are both causal factors. There are plenty of people walking around with the same genetic variation without autism because they didn't have, say, the dose of mercury, or the dose of aluminum, or the combination.

I call people who are most susceptible "Canaries," and I say in the book that they may be the Canaries, but we're all in the cage. We're all sampling all these environmental toxins in our environment, from glyphosate to polyphenol chloride and fire retardants and pesticides aerially sprayed and all these things that are in our environment are likely contributors. It doesn't mean we can throw our hands up in the air and say, "Oh, jeez, everything's causing autism. What are we ever going to do about it?" No, there are things that we can do about it. We can stop putting these toxins into our environment; that would be the first thing to do. Families who have autistic children might do well to look into a clean room for their child. There's a researcher in Pittsburgh named Scott Faber. He and his colleagues put a group of children with autism into a clean room, and interestingly, the younger ones got better very quickly. The older ones got worse first before they got better, and he believes it was because they were getting rid of the toxins, and they became re-intoxicated. The same group found that organic toxins are found to be much higher in kids with autism than in neurotypical kids, and that the severity of behavioral scores are correlated with the serum concentrations of these toxins.

There are ways to reduce toxins in their diet, certainly wash your vegetables, try to eat organic food, and certified organic food, and demand that the certification on organic food remains certified organic. Just try to reduce the amount of artificial chemicals that we put into our body.

DB: Tell us about the Institute for Pure and Applied Knowledge. What are your plans to do with this wonderful organization you formed?

JLW: IPAK. The Institute for Pure and Applied Knowledge, was created to ask questions and do research in the public interest, not in a manner that is meant to derive profit for anyone involved. It's meant to ask and answer questions that may help reduce human pain and suffering. With that as our mission, it's a pretty broad scope. You know, we consume vast quantities of the published literature to try to get a real handle on the state of knowledge on issues. The number one priority for IPAK is to help bring about reform in vaccine research, vaccine safety research in particular, and so we're conducting research studies that are designed to identify proteins in viruses, pathogens, bacteriab and pathogens that may be so similar to human proteins over short stretches of the protein, that it induces autoimmunity, and it activates the immune system against ourselves. We're taking all the autoimmune disorders that we can find that we know of, and looking across all the pathogens for which there's vaccines, and try to find out if there's any epitopes or little protein segments that we might actually be inoculating ourselves against ourselves and inducing autoimmunity. Then of course the genetic information that we just talked about some families might be more prone to those kinds of autoimmune diseases.

There's a great example in Europe of some families that came down with sleep disorders. Some families had been vaccinated by a GSK vaccine, and they came down, across population, with narcolepsy. Other families had other flu vaccine from Novartis. It's the same exact flu strain, but there's something different about the vaccines. One vaccine led to narcolepsy, and GSK's paid out millions of Euros to these families for damages. Molecular mimicry is suspected between epitopes that were found in the GSK vaccine that were not found in the Novartis vaccine, so that's an area of active research for us, not just narcolepsy, but Lupus, multiple sclerosis, ALS, and many other kinds of autoimmune disorders. Type II diabetes is on our table, and just to find out are we making ourselves really, really sick by not stripping the vaccines of these peptides. It's simple to make them safer, really. It's expensive, but it's simple to make them safer.

Some vaccines, they put an attenuation peptide in there, so they have to take a gene out which encodes for protein, and they have to put a spacer gene in that they make up. If that attenuation peptide happens to have a match by chance between any human protein, they're playing Russian Roulette with our autoimmunity.

We also have studies on the levels of aluminum in vaccines. The FDA/CFR limits aluminum dosing to 5 micrograms/kg/day. Hepatitis B gives the average male newborn in the use 74 micrograms/kg in one day, and combined vaccine visits exceed the limit after that. We need to re-visit the schedule from the perspective of pediatric dosing of aluminum, FDA limits, and we may in fact need to consider whether to allow aluminum in vaccines in the first place. Ten percent of aluminum that is injected makes its way into our brains, where it stays for decades. Mercury has a brain half-life of twenty-seven years. What in the world are we thinking, injecting mercury and aluminum into the bodies of babies with developing brains? None of the limits on aluminum are based on safety studies of aluminum injected into mice or rats with developing brains: the safety studies involved dietary aluminum in adult mice. The limit of

850 micrograms per vaccines was not based at all on safety data, but rather on the ability of aluminum to elicit an immune response. And body weight is ignored in the pediatric schedule. The schedule is in violation of FDA/CFR code.

DB: Do you feel comfortable commenting on research papers that disappear that link vaccines and chronic illness?

JLW: You know, we live in a free society, an open society, where ideas should be shared. The marketplace of ideas is a valuable, valuable part of our open society. It's okay to disagree with someone scientifically. If you disagree with them on scientific grounds, then you should have a discussion and a debate. What you're talking about disappearance of papers, you're talking about retraction of papers. The journal all of a sudden decides they're going to pull the paper because there's some expression of concern that is becoming weaponized against studies that point to an association of vaccines and autism. It's censoring in favor of a particular industry agenda. The expressions of concern are often unfounded, and the journals don't reply when you ask them what was the cause for this. They have started to fail to give sufficient detail to assess the ground for retraction, which is atypical, in my experience.

I can also say that the study that Dr. Thompson outed the removal for result showing association is just one of a number of important studies the CDC has relied on to convince everyone that vaccines do not cause autism. I've looked at the other studies, and many of them show signs of concocted results from analysis-to-result. They have routinely rejected positive associations, re-doing the analysis over and over until the association goes away. In one case they had to work at making it go away for four years. Finding positive association was easy; cooking the data to make it go away was more difficult.

What I've chosen to focus on in terms of writing my books hopefully will elevate the discussion such that the demand for ethical behavior on people involved on both sides of the discussion will then be clear.

I haven't really examined the efficacy question problem to the extent that I eventually will, but I'm content for now to say that we need to clean up vaccines. They're terrible, filthy, nasty, toxic concoctions, and they don't have to be. That's the best apart. We can use virus-like particles that are loaded with epitopes that are screened for safety. The expense is well worth it, look at the expense to society, because that work has not been done. I'm sure any parent when offered the current vaccines for free, and cleaner vaccines would pay the additional cost for the cleaner option.

If there's one thing I could successfully convince pharma to do by the end of this year is search for epitopes that match basic myelin proteins, you know? Why in the world would you put an adjuvant in somebody's body at the same time you're putting in an epitope that matches their myelin protein? You could get MS, Parkinson's, all kinds of debilitating, life-altering conditions. We can build our database that will inform families of the risks due to molecular mimicry and inform pharma and so that we can get to the future where we want to be where we have genetic screens for individuals. With an exome sequence, we can know their protein sequence as well. We could tell them: You shouldn't have this vaccine, it has an epitope that's too similar to your protein x. It's very straight-forward. You just have to do the science, it's not difficult to do.

DB: We would all be happy to pay a couple extra dollars to have vaccines that were safer.

JLW: I think parents should really clamor for a safe vaccine. We should also start advocating for safe vaccines and promoting vaccine safety research, and that's what IPAK's all about.

✳ ✳ ✳

I hope you found the information in this chapter helpful. It may have been a tough pill for some of you to swallow. Who wants to believe that one of the most important regulatory agencies out there to protect our children could have committed fraud on a vaccine safety study, especially one as important as looking for a link between vaccines and autism? Who wants to believe that Congress has had this information for almost two years and done nothing, even though the whistleblower CDC scientist wants to come forward and be subpoenaed so he could tell his side of the story? So please don't feel bad about not knowing any of these facts, they are practically hidden from the public every day. Not many people know about the Vaccine Injury Compensation Program until it is past the three year filing deadline, including myself. And almost no parents are told by their pediatricians about how they can report their child's vaccine injury to VAERS, which is the government agency set up to keep track of adverse reactions. In actuality it is the pediatrician's job to do it, but most never seem to, including my son's pediatric office. Unfortunately this is why most people believe that roughly only one to ten percent of vaccine injuries are ever reported to VAERS.

Regarding the ingredient list in vaccines, one could probably write an entire book just to cover and explain each of these substances. So I will leave you with a link to the CDC's vaccine ingredient list which is posted on their website and hopefully will still be there when this book goes to print. Each vaccine is listed with the ingredients that it contains. Here is the link to see the entire list:

http://www.cdc.gov/vaccines/pubs/pinkbook/downloads/appendices/B/excipient-table-2.pdf

An example of an ingredient list of the Varicella vaccine (which is chickenpox) copied from the CDC website: sucrose, phosphate, glutamate, gelatin, monosodium L-glutamate, sodium phosphate dibasic, potassium phosphate monobasic, potassium chloride, sodium phosphate monobasic, potassium chloride, EDTA, residual components of MRC-5 cells including DNA and protein, neomycin, fetal bovine serum, human diploid cell cultures (WI-38), embryonic guinea pig cell cultures, human embryonic lung cultures.

Please note all the different species that are injected with this vaccine, including guinea pig, human diploid cells (aborted fetal cells), and fetal bovine serum. Then there is MSG and antibiotics. The Dtap is even more interesting in some ways in that it includes yeast protein which goes back to what Dr. Baker mentioned earlier about having the immune system overreact to yeast later on. Some of the vaccines listed mention that they contain casein or egg protein, so there is no wonder to me how a vaccine can evoke a food allergy to milk or egg in some children.

I want to state for the record again that I am not trying to talk anyone out of vaccines. It's important that you have all the facts and then make your own decision. You must look over the ingredients the way that you would sit in a supermarket aisle and study a box of cookies or chips to see if you would like to purchase them. We no longer live in a time that we can blindly expect others to do the research and protect us. We must read the literature and studies on Pubmed for ourselves. Pediatricians are under intense pressure not to question anything relating to vaccines. Some doctors have had their careers or license threatened for speaking out. You have to trust yourself to make the best possible decision on this difficult topic. So whether you choose to follow the CDC recommended schedule, create an alternative schedule or not vaccinate at all, remember it is your right to make that decision for your child. You are the parent and only you can know what is best for them! You will also be the only one that must live with the consequences of that decision.

Right now we are going to move on and explore another very important topic, which is an environmental stressor that most people are unfortunately unaware of but come into contact with almost everyday.

CHAPTER SUMMARY

A lead scientist for the CDC came forward and admitted that he and other scientists at the CDC routinely committed fraud on studies designed to test the association between the MMR vaccine and autism.

There is a diverse genetic minority of people that are more susceptible to the toxins in vaccines and more vulnerable to experience an adverse reaction.

Roughly one to two percent of people vaccinated may suffer from a serious vaccine injury.

In 1986, President Ronald Regan, signed the the National Childhood Vaccine Injury Act, which gave pharmaceutical companies protection from people seeking compensation for injuries sustained due to their vaccine products.

The vaccine industry is a multibillion-dollar-a-year business.

Vaccine injuries are under-reported. Estimates are that only one to ten percent of injuries are actually reported.

VAERS (vaccine adverse events reporting system) was set up by the government for reporting vaccine injuries. You do not need to be a doctor or medical professional to report the injury and may do so on your own.

The CDC is not conducting proper studies. Not all individual vaccines, nor the pediatric schedule as it's given in total, have been tested for safety.

There are conflicts of interest occurring where people who may own stock in a company that develops a certain vaccine can also be involved in the decision making on whether or not to bring the particular vaccine onto the pediatric vaccination schedule.

Many people who are called anti-vaccine are not necessarily against vaccines, but would like to have them made safer and be properly tested.

There has been no single gene that has been found to cause autism.

There are more toxins around us today. People may have genes that make them more susceptible to disease, but without the environmental toxic trigger they would not necessarily develop that illness.

We could easily screen vaccines for epitopes that are similar to the ones in our body that could potentially trigger autoimmunity including possibly MS or ALS. There would just be an additional cost associated with it.

Vaccines can and should be made safer.

Chapter 11

GLYPHOSATE AND THE AUTISM EPIDEMIC
with Stephanie Seneff, PhD.

Autism has been growing at exponential rates and so far we have no one singular explanation as to why. Here is what we do know: that the rate of children diagnosed with autism more than thirty years ago was just 1 in 10,000 children. The CDC currently states that the rate is 1 in 68 children; however, we know that number was taken from children born in 2004, which in essence means that it is twelve years behind the times.

One scientist has taken the time to try to figure out and predict how many children will go on to be diagnosed on the autism spectrum that are born this year, in 2017, by taking the CDC's own data and plotting it on a log scale and extending the line forward. So, if the rates of autism have continued to climb at the rate they have been for the past thirty years, then for children born in the year this book is published it will be an astounding 1 in 11 children diagnosed on the autism spectrum. Now if that doesn't frighten you then I really don't know what will. My opinion is that, no matter what your genetics are, you should work as hard as you can to prevent autism given that the odds are so greatly stacked against your child.

Let's try to think of it this way: we know children are being born "pre-polluted" with a great many chemicals, and then you add in the daily environmental assaults that bombard them every day including chemicals and preservatives in our food, pesticides sprayed all around us, electromagnetic radiation coming at us from Wi-Fi practically everywhere, and toxins that can be found in vaccines, our air and water. So, the more things you do to live a clean and healthy life, the further away from the cliff you will be, and it will take a lot more for your child to be pushed over the edge and succumb to an illness. However, if your child is not eating healthy, using toxic products that contain parabens and phthalates everyday then it won't take that much to push them over the edge of the cliff. I hope this analogy of the cliff helps you see the importance of why the choices you make each day not only matter but add up over time. This brings us back to the total load theory, that at some point the body cannot take any more toxins and the immune system eventually implodes and the brain ceases to function properly. And once this happens it can be extremely difficult to get that child back in good health. I can tell you first hand that it takes one thousand times more energy to try to recover them, not to mention the mental anguish, financial hardship, and emotional stress it puts on the entire family. This is why I have worked very hard to bring you the most knowledgeable people in the field to help educate you about all the preventative steps you can take, and this chapter is no different from the others. Of course, it is up to you what you do with this information.

It's clear that we don't know exactly what is causing autism which is why we have to go back to what Dr. Usman explained to us about the precautionary principle and try to discover what has changed so dramatically in the lives of children born after we started to see this sudden increase. One thing we already spoke about was the huge change in the number of vaccines given, which does happen to closely match up with the increase in the number of children being diagnosed with autism. There are still a couple of other things that come to my mind that have also changed in the last couple of decades, one of which we will explore in great detail throughout this chapter. It is a chemical called glyphosate. Most people commonly refer to it as Roundup, which is a formulation made by Monsanto to kill weeds, whose main ingredient is glyphosate. Farmers all over the country spray it on their non-organic produce. Glyphosate can also be found on people's lawns, grassy areas in parks and playgrounds, and other outside recreational areas.

Sadly, the use of glyphosate is pervasive and widespread. Many people are very unaware of its dangers and how much their children are coming into contact with it on a daily basis. I pretty much assume that it is on all food that I buy unless it's labeled organic. Even more upsetting is that many of the California organic wines are turning up with low levels of this chemical when tested due to the fact that when crop planes are spraying the fields the weather conditions can shift where the glyphosate gets sprayed. It's extremely alarming that it is also showing up in high levels in breast milk for women who are conscientious about their diet. People are routinely being told that the product is harmless and dissipates quickly, which is not necessarily true for glyphosate or other pesticides.

One scientist in particular has been studying this issue quite closely and the effects that glyphosate has on people's health. She even goes so far as to say that it is the driving force behind the current autism epidemic. In this chapter, we will explore the detrimental effects of glyphosate and how it contributes to disease, paying specific attention to autism.

Stephanie Seneff is a senior research scientist at MIT's Computer Science and Artificial Intelligence Laboratory and also holds four degrees from the institute, including a BS in biology, and MS, EE, and PhD degrees in electrical engineering and computer science. She has recently been focusing her attention on the important role that environmental toxins and nutrition play in developing disease. Stephanie's research findings have been published in over two hundred peer-reviewed papers that have appeared in many different scientific journals. She has also presented her research at conferences all around the world as well as in this country including at a Congressional hearing. Stephanie has been kind enough to share with us everything she knows about this widely used environmental toxin and the grave consequences it can have on our health.

DB: What is glyphosate?

SS: Glyphosate is the active ingredient in the pervasive herbicide Roundup, which is considered to be non-toxic to humans and therefore very widely used. It's the herbicide that's used on the GMO Roundup-Ready crops, and these are the core crops of the processed food industry, so it's very pervasive in our food supply at this point. And it has not been well monitored in the food, and it has not been assessed adequately in tests to see if it's actually safe to humans as is claimed.

DB: How widely do you feel that it is being used right now?

SS: The use of glyphosate has been going up exponentially ever since about the late 1990s when they introduced the GMO Roundup-Ready crops. This is the corn, soy, canola, sugar beets, alfalfa, cotton, and tobacco that are all GMO Roundup-Ready. They are now more and more commonly spraying Roundup on other crops that are not GMO as a desiccant right before harvest. This is a very serious problem, because glyphosate is showing up in high concentrations in wheat, and of course sugar cane is sprayed right before harvest. Sugar beets are also GMO Roundup-Ready, and of course, high fructose corn syrup comes from corn, so all of the sugars will have glyphosate in them. It's also in beans. I was very surprised to find high levels of glyphosate in hummus, because chickpeas are sprayed right before the harvest. I believe peanuts are too, and I think that may be a major factor in the peanut allergy epidemic that we are seeing today.

So, the usage of glyphosate has gone up astronomically over the past two decades. Part of the reason is because the GMO weeds are becoming resistant to glyphosate, especially among the GMO crops, so they're having to use a higher concentration of glyphosate to actually maintain control of the weeds. Every year it gets worse, and it's actually becoming to the point of collapse. Right now, they've started to introduce new chemicals that have glyphosate plus, so glyphosate plus 2,4-D or glyphosate plus dicamba or some other herbicide on top of the glyphosate to help to control those weeds that have become resistant. So we're reaching a point almost where glyphosate is no longer useful.

DB: Should people who are spraying Roundup on their lawn be worried that it might be harmful? I know a lot of people think when they spray it that a couple hours later it's fine, or when it rains it will get washed away. Is this true? Does it disappear quickly?

SS: That's not true at all. In fact, glyphosate can survive for years in certain conditions, depending upon the soil conditions. Monsanto has claimed that it disappears in about two weeks, but that is actually turning out not to be true. And in fact it's been shown that glyphosate that's washed off into the sea will stay in the ocean for a year. It also really depends upon whether there are microbes in the soil that can break it down, and if there aren't it is actually very difficult to break down. There are very few microbes that know how to break down glyphosate, so it sticks around, and it also changes into other products that may be even more toxic than glyphosate itself.

DB: How is glyphosate different from other pesticides that have been used?

SS: My recent research with Anthony Samsel over the past year has been remarkable, because I believe we have hit pay dirt in terms of understanding why glyphosate is insidiously, cumulatively toxic. And it's not a unique property of glyphosate, because glufosinate is similar. Glyphosate is a glycine molecule with additional material stuck onto the nitrogen. Glycine is an amino acid, one of the coding amino acids. They go into the proteins of the body with the DNA code. So Anthony and I both believe that glyphosate goes into proteins by mistake during protein synthesis. The synthesis machinery makes a mistake and puts glyphosate in place of glycine. If this is true, it is very serious, because it means that throughout your body, various proteins will get glyphosate in random places where it shouldn't be, and it can completely ruin a protein's ability to do its job if it happens to show up in a critical place in that protein.

It can also make the protein very difficult to break down, and so that protein will stick around and become allergenic, and I think this is what's happening with many of the foods. We have all these allergies today to casein in milk, gluten in wheat, and peanut allergy that I mentioned before. I believe these allergies and the epidemic that we're seeing is due to the fact that glyphosate is getting into those proteins. All of those foods can be expected to be exposed to glyphosate. It gets into the protein, and then the protein resists being broken down, and that's how your immune system reacts to these foreign proteins. And then you go through something called molecular mimicry where it can attack your own body's proteins and cause disease. It can cause autoimmune disease like Lupus, chronic fatigue syndrome, and even autism is considered by many to be an autoimmune disease, and I believe this is what's happening there.

DB: How is it getting into the casein protein that's in milk? Is it because the cows are eating the glyphosate from their feed?

SS: That's exactly right. Most cows today are fed GMO Roundup-Ready corn and soy feed. You know there is also a GMO Roundup-Ready grass, but I do not understand how much and to what extent that's being used. That is terrifying to me. If they start using GMO Roundup-Ready grass and spray it with glyphosate, and then have cows grazing on the grass. I rely on grass-fed beef. I will not eat the beef that comes from a confined animal feeding operation. You know those cows are fed toxic food that's loaded with glyphosate, in the corn and the soy feed that they get. Monsanto themselves have shown in a study that Anthony Samsel has that glyphosate showed up in the milk. I believe it was goats that they used, but you know any kind of mammalian species that produces milk is going to push that glyphosate out into the milk. That means humans as well, of course. It's not just that the glyphosate is in the food as a loose molecule. The glyphosate is intimately bound into the protein, so it's very difficult to get rid of it under those circumstances.

DB: How else is glyphosate so dangerous, besides getting into the protein?

SS: Well originally Anthony Samsel and I wrote a paper talking about glyphosate's effect on the gut microbes. Monsanto argues that glyphosate is pretty harmless to humans, because we don't have the biological pathway that it disrupts in plants, and that pathway is called the shikimate pathway. Unfortunately, our gut microbes do have that shikimate pathway, and they use it to produce very essential molecules that our own cells cannot produce for themselves precisely because they don't have that pathway. So we rely on our gut microbes to provide certain nutrients for us using the pathway that glyphosate interrupts. If the microbes in the gut are exposed to glyphosate then these nutrients become deficient. They are specifically the aromatic amino acids: phenylalanine, tryptophan, and tyrosine. These are also building blocks of proteins, just like glycine. Those are also called amino acids that go into protein called coding. But they are also precursors to a lot of really important nutrients and molecules in the body, biologically active molecules, such as serotonin, melatonin, melanin, thyroid hormone, various B vitamins, vitamin K, all these things come from the shikimate pathway. You can expect them to be deficient if the microbes aren't able to produce these amino acids.

The microbes are also harmed, because another thing that glyphosate does is it's an extremely strong chelating agent. It binds very tightly to specific metals that are called +2 cations. Things like zinc, manganese, magnesium, calcium, molybdenum, and cobalt are all really important nutrients. These minerals are often catalysts for various enzymes in our body. If those minerals are bound tightly to glyphosate, then we become mineral deficient. And I've also written about how glyphosate disrupts the body's transport mechanisms for these minerals, so that the minerals can become both simultaneously toxic and deficient at the same time.

This is happening, for example, with iron. It's very clear to me that I'm seeing around the world, as countries adopt a western diet, they get into a situation where there's both iron toxicity and anemia. The iron is not getting to where it needs to go, and if the iron is not being carefully ushered during transport, it becomes toxic in the blood, and it can cause a lot of damage to the blood vessels.

DB: Can glyphosate be passed along in breast milk?

SS: Monsanto executives have claimed that glyphosate isn't in milk, but they don't seem to realize or they just don't know that these studies were done. I want to mention that Zen Honeycutt had human breast milk tested, and she found I think a third of the women tested had glyphosate present in their breast milk. The highest level was 1,600 times higher than the upper limit allowed in water in Europe, which was in the mother's breast milk. And these women who were being tested were mostly pretty conscientious about trying to avoid GMO food, so I suspect that other women would have even higher levels of glyphosate in their breast milk. So Zen Honeycutt of Moms Across America did find glyphosate in breast milk, human breast milk.

DB: So interesting, all those things you had listed a little while ago are all the problems we have with our children that have autism. They are deficient in B vitamins, melatonin, amino acids, serotonin, and have issues with their thyroid, literally everything you just named.

SS: I really think glyphosate is the reason for the autism epidemic. It's not the only thing that can cause autism, since it existed before glyphosate was present. But it is what's causing the epidemic.

DB: More so than the damage from vaccines?

SS: The vaccines are working together with glyphosate. The vaccines, of course, are providing nasty metals like aluminum and mercury, then glyphosate is making those metals much more toxic than they would otherwise be. The two are working synergistically together to cause harm. Glyphosate is making the vaccines much more likely to cause autism. Of course, there's also the issue of glyphosate in the vaccines, which we haven't gotten to yet but that is something that has me absolutely alarmed.

I believe that glyphosate is getting into the vaccines, and in fact, several vaccines have been tested and have come out positive for glyphosate. This is just absolutely terrifying to think about injecting glyphosate into the child's body. You pass all the protective barriers, one hundred percent of the glyphosate gets in. It's probably already embedded in the proteins in the vaccine, and those proteins are specifically there to cause an immune reaction. So when you get in a situation where a glyphosate contaminated protein in a vaccine causes an immune reaction that ends up being an autoimmune attack on the brain through molecular mimicry. I think that is really the key story that I see causing autism.

DB: So let me understand how you think it's getting into the vaccine. Is it getting into the proteins by the way of how it's being made? So if it's made on human embryonic cells or if it's cultured on monkey kidney cells. Is that where it's getting in?

SS: Well in fact there's a couple of ways. Some of these vaccines are a live virus that's grown, for example on mediums such as fetal bovine serum, so that's the blood of a baby cow or calf. Fetal bovine serum of the calf is of course exposed to glyphosate. Even in the womb they are exposed to glyphosate, because there's so much glyphosate in the calf's mother, the cow. So the live virus being grown on a glyphosate contaminated medium is going to take up the glyphosate, and just like humans incorporates it into the viral proteins.

One example is that hemagglutinin is produced by the measles virus, and hemagglutinin is the key protein that you need to react to in order to obtain immunity against measles. The whole point of the vaccine is to get your immune system to recognize hemagglutinin and develop specific antibodies to it. I believe what happens in the case of autism is that that hemagglutinin that's in the measles virus protein is synthesized in the presence of glyphosate, so it has glyphosate in the protein itself. This makes that hemagglutinin extremely difficult to break down.

Glyphosate also sets up leaky barriers. It sets up leaky gut barrier and leaky brain barrier, so this is going to allow that hemagglutinin to get into the brain. And hemagglutinin happens to have a peptide sequence that closely resembles a sequence in myelin basic protein, which is an important protein in the myelin sheath. When the myelin basic protein gets attacked by the immune system, because it looks like the protein of the peptide sequence in the hemagglutinin, then you get an attack of the nerve fibers in the brain. This will really cause trouble in terms of the ability for the neurons to deliver a signal along the axons that travel long distance. For example, the eyes: all of the communication that goes on with the world requires these long axons that are going to be damaged by the immune system attacking them because they resemble the peptide sequence in the hemagglutinin that was fed to the child through the vaccine.

DB: Could something like MS be triggered in this way?

SS: Absolutely. In fact, Anthony Samsel and I have a new paper that's been accepted by a journal and will hopefully soon appear online as an Open-Access paper. We talk about the MMR vaccine in particular, which had the highest concentration of glyphosate among the vaccines that we tested. The MMR vaccine also causes many more adverse reactions today than it used to. I've looked at the VAERS database, the Vaccine Adverse Event Reporting System going back from the beginning in 1990 when the data were first being collected. If you look statistically at the types of events that are occurring today, like in the last decade versus in the 1990s, you see many more severe adverse reactions today than there used to be for the same vaccine. So there's a puzzle as to why is this vaccine much more toxic now than it used to be? I think the answer lies in both the fact that glyphosate's in the air, our food, and water. The kids are being exposed to it, so they're more vulnerable to problems with the vaccine. Then on top of that, the actual glyphosate in the vaccine is probably really critical to throw it over the top and cause this acute reaction, such as anaphylactic shock or seizures. Subsequently the child slowly regresses into autism, because of this autoimmune attack on the nerve fibers in the brain.

DB: So what other vaccines did you find glyphosate in?

SS: The flu vaccine. I personally have never had a flu vaccine, and I don't intend to ever get one. I think that the flu vaccine is definitely not worth the risk, even if it didn't have glyphosate in it. As long as you keep yourself healthy, the flu is not going to present much of a problem for you. If you get the flu and you're in bed for a week it will strengthen your immune system to actually get the disease. Whereas the vaccine has a risk. Many of the flu vaccines still have mercury, and the mercury is going to be synergistically toxic with the glyphosate as well.

It was interesting, because we did not find it in vaccines, which were not prepared as a live virus grown on fetal bovine serum and which did not have gelatin. So, gelatin is another critical factor to provide the glyphosate in the vaccine. Gelatin is derived from the collagen of cows and pigs, derived from their bones and ligaments. That's where you get the gelatin. Collagen is the most common protein in the body. You know, it's in all your connective tissue. It's a really important protein, since twenty-five percent of the protein in your body is collagen, and collagen is incredibly loaded up on glycine. Twenty-five percent of the amino acids in collagen are glycine residues, so this means that collagen has a tremendous opportunity to get glyphosate substituting for glycine in the protein. In fact, Anthony tested collagen and gelatin. He found high levels of glyphosate in both of these sources, so it makes sense that the vaccines that include gelatin, which are many of them, will be contaminated. And we confirmed that that is the case.

We have not tested Gardasil, and I'm very eager to find out whether Gardasil has glyphosate, because looking at how it's manufactured, I would it expect it to. Gardasil is interesting, because what they've done with Gardasil is they've taken the proteins that are produced by the viruses, the HPV virus, those specific proteins that need to become the source of your immunity. Your body is going to react to those proteins. You will get immune sensitivity to them, and then you're going to have resistance supposedly to this HPV virus. Those proteins are incorporated into the genome of yeast cells, and those yeast cells are then encouraged to grow and produce these foreign proteins through the genomic modification. It's a GMO yeast that produces these HPV proteins, and they feed the yeast galactose, which is derived from milk presumably from cows. I would expect that is contaminated with glyphosate. Then I would predict that the Gardasil vaccine would also have proteins with glyphosate embedded in them, because of this process through the yeast producing the protein.

DB: This GMO yeast you're talking about is very scary.

SS: Yes, it is very scary. As I look more into how vaccines are made, it just amazes me. You know, we have so much discussion about GMO foods and how disturbed we are that we're eating these GMO foods, but we're not paying attention to how they're making these vaccines. It is really bizarre science. It is science fiction practically, and I just don't feel they've done enough studies to confirm that this stuff is safe, even irrespective of the glyphosate.

DB: Could you please explain to people about this synergistic effect that glyphosate has in the presence of other toxins?

SS: Well, yes it's because glyphosate binds to metals like mercury and aluminum, which are both metals in the vaccine. So if there's glyphosate in the vaccine, I would predict that the glyphosate would bind to those metals, and that the combination would be extremely toxic. In fact, I wrote a paper together with colleagues, about glyphosate escorting aluminum to the brain. Glyphosate carries the metal to what they call the terminal watershed of the vascular system, so to the places where the blood equilibrates with other fluids. So for example, the kidneys, where you have the urine, the blood equilibrates with the urine. These are the most acidic environments of the vascular system, and so that's where in that acidic environment, glyphosate will carry that metal into those places.

So this happens with the urine, but more critically the pineal gland in the brain stem, where the blood equilibrates with the cerebral spinal fluid or with the saliva, and that's also an acidic environment. This is sort of still theoretical, but it makes sense from a scientific standpoint, and then it lets go of it, releasing that toxic metal, as well as then the glyphosate itself becoming toxic at that point once the two of them separate. They both become very toxic to the pineal gland, and, of course, this is going to disrupt sleep, because the pineal gland produces melatonin, and as I mentioned, melatonin is a product of the shikimate pathway, so that's another double hit. The pineal gland will be disrupted, so that it can't function, which will then lead to sleep disturbances, and sleep disturbances are going up in this country exponentially in step with the rise in the use of glyphosate on core crops.

DB: And then tell us how glyphosate can hurt our DNA?

SS: Absolutely. There are in vitro studies that they've done that have shown that it causes these certain changes in the genome that are precursors of cancer, sort of moving towards carcinogenic. Anthony and I wrote about this in a paper that we have published on this idea of glyphosate substituting for glycine. There are proteins that are concerned with

DNA repair. So as the synthesis process is going on, if a mistake is made, there are these proteins that their job is to fix it, and these proteins know how to fix that mistake. But those proteins depend critically upon essential glycines to do that job. So if those glycines get displaced by glyphosate then those proteins won't work, the DNA repair won't happen, and you'll have a much higher risk, and this will lead you to cancer through DNA mutations. It's really the precursor to cancers. Also there are correlations. Nancy Swanson has done a lot of investigation looking at different diseases and certain cancers such as bladder cancer, pancreatic cancer, and thyroid cancer in particular. Nancy showed from US data that they're all going up very dramatically, exponentially in recent times in step with an exact match really with the exponential growth in the use of glyphosate. So I'm suspecting it's causing at least those three cancers, and I also believe it's causing prostate cancer, breast cancer, and ovarian cancer. The liver and the kidney are very stressed by glyphosate, so it's causing liver and kidney cancer. Probably also brain cancer, certainly Non-Hodgkin lymphoma, and leukemia.

Below are two graphs that show the correlation in the rise of bladder and thyroid cancer with an increase in the use of glyphosate on soy and corn.

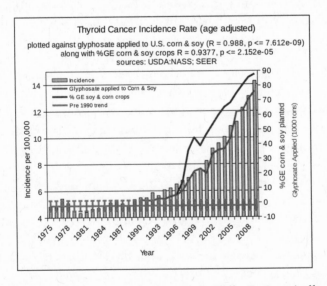

Figure 9 from Swanson NL, Leu A, Abrahamson J, Wallet B. Genetically engineered crops, glyphosate, and the deterioration of health in the United States of America. J. Organic Systems 2014; 9: 6-37. Reproduced with permission from author.

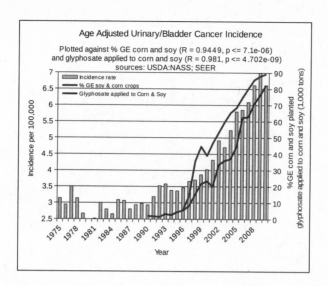

Figure 10 from Swanson NL, Leu A, Abrahamson J, Wallet B. Genetically engineered crops, glyphosate, and the deterioration of health in the United States of America. J. Organic Systems 2014; 9: 6-37. Reproduced with permission from author.

SS: Glyphosate accumulates in the bone marrow, and the bone marrow is where the blood cells come out of and mature. There are these precursor cells that come out of the bone marrow and mature into white blood cells, which are really the immune cells, immune system cells. Those cells are going to come out of that bone marrow already loaded up with glyphosate, and that will disrupt their function, and lead to cancer as well as other problems.

DB: I think most people don't understand that if they're eating anything that's not organic, there is a good chance that glyphosate is on that food item.

SS: There are many food items that have glyphosate on them, and we're starting to get a picture of exactly which ones. There's a man in Canada named Tony Mitra, who is an activist in Canada. He's really great, and he has managed to get the Canadian government, very recently to give him a list of thousands of samples of different foods that they've tested for glyphosate, and these foods come from other places too. It's mostly Canada and the US, but they also have data from other countries. He's been tabulating all of this data and analyzing it. This is how I found out that there are very high levels in chickpeas, which I hadn't necessarily suspected. So you can start to know which foods are especially problematic.

Interestingly, the Germans found glyphosate in beers they tested, I don't know, maybe twelve different kinds of beer, and they found glyphosate in all of them. Zen Honeycutt tested wines in California, and she found glyphosate contamination in all of them, including the biodynamics, which had lower levels, but not zero. So even organic is not necessarily one hundred percent certain to not have glyphosate in it. It's just that organic usually has a lot less on average than non-organic.

DB: Let me make sure I understand one thing. What happens is the glyphosate gets in in place of the glycine?

SS: That is certainly one thing, and I think that is in my opinion the most important thing that's happening. It's not generally known if this is happening. We haven't yet proven it. Anthony and I have enormous amounts of circumstantial evidence, and we're moving towards proving it. Anthony is a chemist, and he's working on it. It's a problem that people are finding very inconsistent results when they test proteins for glyphosate. This is because if you don't get it out of that protein, then you won't see it. That's what's really insidious. So you could have a protein sample that you test for glyphosate, and it comes out negative. You think: oh good this doesn't have glyphosate, but it's not true if it's embedded in the protein. Unless you do a chemical pre-processing step that disassembles that protein, the method will fail to detect the glyphosate that's in it.

Anthony has been doing research to try to figure out how to deal with these problems with the proteins. Hopefully he'll come up with a solution that's pretty reliable to actually know that the glyphosate is in the protein through the test.

We're in a difficult situation and we need more science. It's ridiculous to me that this chemical is so pervasive especially in the US We are exposed to more glyphosate in this country than any other country in the world with the possible exception of Brazil. We're very big on processed foods, and glyphosate is all over the processed foods, and I think that's the reason why the United States has by far the most expensive health care system in the world with very little to show for it, in terms of poor performance.

Among the industrialized world, we are the last. We are the worst in terms of death on the first day of life, and we also have a very poor life expectancy compared to most of the other industrialized nations. We spend huge amounts of money, and we don't get reward for that money. We're not seeing success in terms of the treatments. We've got so many people that are so sick. We've got opiate epidemics, because people are overdosing on painkillers. I think because of glyphosate getting into the collagen and other places, but the collagen in particular. If you get glyphosate into the collagen of your joints, the joints don't work properly, and you're going to get a lot of joint pain. You get back pain. You get knee pain. I mean all of these different pains that people are experiencing I think are due to contamination of glyphosate in the collagen.

We're getting it in food. We're getting it in vaccines. It's probably in our water as well. People are probably breathing it, if they live near farms where it's being sprayed. And, of course, kids are coming into contact with it on the playground. Even in the home, a mother could be pregnant applying glyphosate to the weeds not realizing she's breathing in these fumes, and it causes her child to be deformed. It's really scary. Safety studies for glyphosate exposure to pregnant women are basically non-existent, since glyphosate is falsely presumed to be nontoxic to humans.

DB: So let's talk about why GMOs make it possible to spray even more glyphosate and why this is such a huge problem.

SS: It is actually very interesting to me how the GMO engineering is done, specifically for glyphosate. Among all the GMOs, the two most popular ones are glyphosate resistance, and then the Bt gene, which builds a code for the protein that makes the insecticide right into the crop. The Bt corn is one, for example, and the Bt cotton. The other really popular GMO is a reengineering of the gene that codes for an enzyme in the shikimate pathway that glyphosate disrupts in plants and microbes. They had identified that this enzyme is critical for the failure of a plant when it's exposed to glyphosate. It disrupts this enzyme, called EPSP synthase, which actually has a glycine at the active site. There are at least three different microbes, bacteria that have come up with an elegant solution to protect themselves from glyphosate, which is to get rid of that glycine! They actually mutated their gene, so that that glycine is now alanine instead. Alanine is very similar to glycine. It has an extra methyl group, but it's not glycine and therefore it doesn't get glyphosate substituted for it, and then that totally solves the problem of glyphosate not making that enzyme work. So three different microbes figured that out, and the GMO that they put into the plants is borrowed from one of those clever microbes. They took that very same EPSP synthase gene from that microbe with the alanine instead of glycine, and they put that gene into the plant so that the plant can now make this enzyme impervious to glyphosate disruption, because it has an alanine there instead of glycine.

Of course, that plant is not completely immune to glyphosate. Glyphosate does damage that plant, but not in this direct way of that particular enzyme. That enzyme is safe, and that is really a critical enzyme that causes immediate stress for the plant. There's more sort of generic stress everywhere as the plant also incorporates glyphosate into its various proteins. The plant is certainly not as healthy as it would have been without the glyphosate exposure, but it's sufficiently healthy to be able to grow and produce food.

DB: Tell us about how glyphosate gives the farmer the ability to spray more on the plant and why this is a problem?

SS: It's really just because you no longer have to be careful to spray the glyphosate only on the weed and not on the plant. It used to be that you had to really be very particular about where you put the glyphosate to kill the weeds. If you can make your plant resistant, you can just fly in the airplane over the field and just spray the glyphosate everywhere all over the plant. The plant soaks up the glyphosate and incorporates it into its own tissues, but it doesn't die, so that's why the glyphosate ends up in the food.

DB: Do you think that genetically modified foods are safe for people to eat in general?

SS: I don't. I mean I don't know as much about GMOs as I do about glyphosate, and I think they're harder to understand, since there are a lot of unknowns. We're playing God, but we really don't know enough to know what's really going on with them. So I could predict that some absolutely bizarre things could be happening that we're not aware of with those GMOs, because it's extremely abnormal biology, and that just really worries me.

Even when they test the GMOs, one thing they say is that the GMO crop is substantially equivalent to the non-GMO crop, meaning that the proteins and all of the different molecules that it produces are sort of the same as the non-GMO crop. They haven't necessarily proven this. They haven't done adequate research to prove that, but that's what they claim. But when they actually compare the GMO with the non-GMO, they actually don't apply glyphosate to the GMO crop, which is really crazy, because the glyphosate is the whole point of the GMO. And if it is exposed to glyphosate, it's definitely going to change its metabolism and will change the different ratios of the things that it produces. So by testing it without actually exposing it to glyphosate, they're not testing it in the environment in which it's actually used. I'm just shocked that they don't consider it necessary to expose it to glyphosate when they're trying to access whether it is in fact substantially equivalent.

DB: Not shocking to me at all. It's kind of like how they use a placebo of aluminum or mercury when they're testing vaccines.

SS: Exactly. I was so shocked when I first heard that. I just almost could not believe it. It's brilliant, because you can protect people from the knowledge that the stuff is toxic by simply exposing the placebo group to the same toxin.

DB: Babies are being born with something like two hundred chemicals in their cord blood. Do you think it's possible that glyphosate is something that could be passed onto an offspring?

SS: I absolutely do. I think the mother is probably pushing the glyphosate in through the placenta, and it's getting into the child before it's born.

DB: You came up with a pretty alarming statistic that predicts 1 in 2 children will have autism by the year 2032. Can you tell me about this?

SS: The prediction was really just based on the trends for autism, which were exponential growth, and then just projecting that. Exponential growth is actually easy to predict for the future, because you just plot it on a log scale, and it becomes a straight line. If it is exponential, it will be a straight line on a log scale. In fact the autism growth is exponential, so you can just extend that straight line into the future and just read off the numbers. It's very easy to predict if it continues to be exponential growth as it has been. In 2032, fifty percent of the kids, eighty percent of the boys born will end up on the autism spectrum, if this trend continues.

Now, this past year it's really interesting when you look at the numbers. You're probably aware of this, because it was exponential growth really right up until 2015. The CDC does this estimate based on twelve-year-olds. They're looking specifically at kids who are twelve years old. In between they do a survey, and they just call different phone numbers and ask people how many kids they have with autism in their family. They count up the numbers after doing a survey. So it was a survey year in 2015, and it was above the exponential growth.

So when you're talking twelve-year-olds, you've got to take another extra twelve years to get to the kids being born. You're not even looking at the kids being born today, so you have to actually extend that curve out twelve years to say children being born today.

The number the CDC released for twelve-year-olds in 2016 was exactly the same as the number in 2014: 1 in 68. I personally don't believe it. Exponential growth for three decades doesn't just suddenly come to a halt! I think they are manipulating the diagnoses—putting autism kids into another category like pervasive developmental delay or a social disorder. If you look at the data that California provides from it's public school system, exponential growth has continued right up through 2016.

Here is Stephanie's linear log scale, which shows the exponential growth based on the CDC's own data:

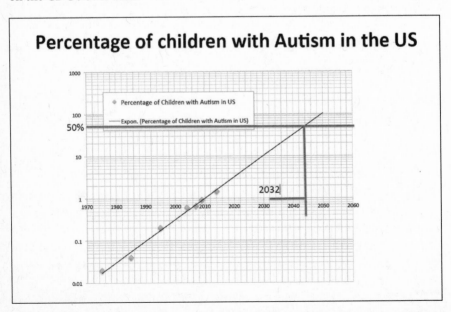

Percentage of children with Autism in the US

DB: Do you think people understand that it doesn't reflect the present day when the CDC releases its autism number to the public?

SS: People don't realize that. I have talked to a clinician informally. She was a person who worked with autistic kids, and her belief from her own impression was that she thinks that up to 1 in 10 or 1 in 11 boys born today are ending up on the spectrum. I'm so worried about the young boys. I see so many kids already with different food issues and failure to thrive. There are a lot of problems going on including all these food allergies and problems like eczema and asthma. The kids are just really hurting today. It's really sad to see kids with ADD and they're drugging them up in the school system. Not just with autism, but all these other things as well.

DB: And then the other thing that I was curious about is why we did not see a big decrease in autism the year that they took the mercury out?

SS: Aluminum. They increased the requirements of aluminum containing vaccines simultaneously with the removal of the mercury.

And of course, glyphosate was also going up very rapidly at that time. That was when they had first introduced those GMO Roundup Ready crops, and those were really taking off right around that time.

DB: What is it about pesticides that contribute so much to autism?

SS: Well, glyphosate in particular, and I've written a lot about that, and I talk a lot about sulfur. I don't know if you're aware of that, but I really believe that sulfate deficiency is a key factor in autism and in many other modern diseases. Glyphosate is an absolute train wreck for sulfate, for sulfur in general, but sulfate in particular. Sulfate is SO_4-2, so it's a sulfur and oxygen. It's one sulfur, four oxygens and negative two charge. That sulfate is a super important molecule in the body, and a molecule that, like iron, is difficult to transport and really important to establish all throughout your body.

There are sulfate ions that are attached to the sugars that are in the, what's called the glycocalyx. It's a part of the blood vessel, the lining of the blood vessels all throughout your body is this glycocalyx, and that glycocalyx has sulfate sprinkled throughout it. And if there aren't enough sulfates, then you get into lots of trouble with respect to both blood and gut barriers being compromised. So things can get in. Things can get out, and your immune cells get dysfunctional. So you have a weakened immune system, and you're unable to clear cellular debris. And then when molecules get damaged, for example, from oxidation damage or from sugar damage, they can't be recycled. If you don't have enough sulfate, it becomes difficult to break them down and reassemble them into fresh, healthy molecules. All those things are problematic, and they're all problematic in autism.

DB: A few of the practitioners talk about the sulfation pathway and how much it affects a child when it is impaired. Can you explain how glyphosate directly affects it?

SS: There is an enzyme called sulfite oxidase, which has essential glycines and if those are displaced by glyphosate, the enzyme will totally be busted. Sulfite oxidase also depends on molybdenum, which is one of those minerals that glyphosate chelates. So you can expect it to be disrupted. Sulfite oxidase is how you make sulfate, so you know there is going to be a problem. There are also sulfotranferases that are essential and have essential glycines. All of these proteins that are involved in managing sulfur are disrupted by glyphosate.

DB: So what do you think is causing this huge rise in autism?

SS: Glyphosate plus the vaccines, and, of course, also nutrient deficiencies. I think the food is critical, all the processed food, which are loaded up on glyphosate and deficient in certain minerals and vitamins. Then there is a disrupted gut microbiome, which is huge for children with autism. I think gut dysbiosis is a huge issue. More and more people are realizing that autistic kids have problems with their gut. It makes sense, because the glyphosate is killing off the beneficial bacteria and allowing the pathogens to overgrow, and of course you have the mineral deficiency problem too, because of glyphosate. And you have issues with absorption of things like cobalamin which is vitamin B12, because of glyphosate. It's really messing up a lot of things in the body that's causing it not to be healthy.

There is this whole methylation pathway too, which is actually very tightly connected to the sulfation pathway. They include all the sulfur containing amino acids like methionine, cysteine, homocysteine, and taurine. All of those amino acids that contain sulfur are problematic in autism. Methionine is the source of the methyl for the methylation pathway, but methionine can also be converted into cysteine then homocysteine and then sulfate. So methionine deficiency is another key factor. In fact, glyphosate has been shown to deplete methionine in plants, so you can expect it to also deplete methionine in animals.

I looked into it and there is an enzyme that is a rate-limiting enzyme in the synthesis of methionine, which has been shown to be suppressed by glyphosate in E. coli. These are bacteria in the gut, so what this means is that methionine synthesis is impaired in the gut in the presence of glyphosate. The gut microbes make the methionine for us, but they can't. So it's another one of those nutrients that are affected, negatively affected, by the glyphosate. And when there's not enough methionine, then there's not enough methylation pathway, and there's not enough sulfate, because methionine is a source of both of those.

DB: Is glyphosate a much bigger problem for you if you have an MTHFR genetic break?

SS: Exactly, and that's what you're seeing, I think, with all the genes. I think that it's very interesting to look at the various genes that are associated with autism and connect them up to pathways that are impaired by glyphosate. I think that's what is happening is that, if you've already got a bit of impairment in that gene, then you are that much more susceptible to the damage that glyphosate causes to that same gene, that same protein.

DB: What things would you do to end or slow down the epidemic of autism if it were up to you?

SS: Obviously organic diet. I would like to get glyphosate banned worldwide. That would be my number one goal. I like the fact that organic is really booming in this country. I think organic produce availability is growing exponentially, which is really awesome. So eating organic is very important, and, of course, I think eating foods that are rich in sulfur is important, because of the sulfur deficiency problem. And then eating probiotics, and I like it to be foods that are naturally probiotics, so things like yogurt, cheese, sauerkraut, and kimchi. Apple cider vinegar, which would be natural unprocessed, so that it has the microbes in it. Both sauerkraut and apple cider vinegar have a bacterium called acetobacter. And acetobacter is on that very short list of microbes that can metabolize glyphosate. So I'm suspecting that one is especially beneficial for that reason, that you can actually clear the glyphosate by letting these bacteria break it down. It's really great. So I very much recommend sauerkraut and apple cider vinegar.

I believe in eating foods that are rich in animal fat and cholesterol, but, of course, you have to be very careful that they are healthy. For example, fish is really good, and I think that's mainly because of the taurine. Taurine is a really important sulfur containing amino acid that fish have a lot of, but with fish you're risking mercury. These days you have to worry about making sure that you're buying the healthiest form of the particular food that you're trying to buy. Grass fed beef is great assuming that the grass isn't GMO Roundup-Ready grass. I certainly hope they haven't put that out there yet! I know that it exists, and I just don't know how widely it's been adopted.

I mentioned fish, but scallops, oysters, clams, all those shell fish are extremely nutritious. They are very rich in micro-nutrients, minerals, vitamins, and, of course, they also have cholesterol, which is actually very important. I think a cholesterol deficiency can contribute to autism, because the brain is five percent of the body's mass and twenty-five percent of the body's cholesterol. The brain loves cholesterol, and it needs cholesterol to be healthy. If you're eating a low cholesterol, low fat diet, that's not good. When a mother is pregnant with a baby, she needs cholesterol and healthy fats, which in my opinion is saturated fats. This is something that is in discord with what the modern, nutritional experts are speaking about. They claim that saturated fats are bad for you, but that is not true. The trans fats are really terrible, but saturated fats are healthy. They actually cannot be oxidized. They're already fully oxidized, so they don't suffer from oxidation damage. It's the oxidation damage on unsaturated fats that's causing fats to be a problem.

I would say number one, making sure the child is eating a one-hundred-percent organic diet to the extent that that's possible. Number two, eating a diet that's rich in saturated animal fat and cholesterol, but maybe being very careful to choose high quality products such as grass-fed beef and organic eggs. Eating foods that have live probiotics, and I mentioned the sauerkraut, yogurt, cheese. Those kinds of things will help to renew the gut microbes and help to maintain a healthy gut, which is so important in autism and also in general health.

Also getting outside in the sunlight without sunscreen and without sunglasses, so the body can use it to make sulfate. The sunlight can really help to boost the immune system. And of course, the immune system is the crucial thing. And to make the immune system healthy, by not piling the child full of vaccines, but by keeping the child in a healthy environment where they're not exposed to toxic chemicals.

Try to avoid foods that are mostly just empty calories. Eat lots of vegetables. I really like green vegetables especially the cruciferous vegetables, which are high in sulfur, and also onion, garlic, ginger, and various herbs. Cruciferous vegetables include broccoli, cauliflower, Brussels sprouts and cabbage. Herbs are also really good. They're good as sulfate transporters, because they have the polyphenols and flavonoids that can actually transport sulfate, so again, all of this fits into the sulfate deficiency problem.

Another thing is fulvic acid and humic acid, which are organic matter from the soil. A very interesting study on cows showed that the cows were contaminated with glyphosate and they were sick. They measured the glyphosate in the urine. They fed the cows fulvic acid, humic acid, sauerkraut juice and bentonite clay, I believe, as a treatment program and then they showed that the urinary glyphosate levels went down after this treatment and the cows' health improved. So this was really an exciting paper that showed how you can help to restore the health of cows exposed to high levels of glyphosate.

DB: Do you think glyphosate has been studied enough for safety? Have there been a lot of studies?

SS: The studies are woefully inadequate. I think it's ridiculous that they have allowed this product to be so pervasive in the food supply, the water supply, and without sufficient studies to confirm that it's safe.

DB: What did the World Health Organization recently say in regards to glyphosate?

SS: There was a recent study and the World Health Organization's International Agency for Research on Cancer said that glyphosate is a probable carcinogen. Interestingly, California picked up on that. I don't know if you're aware of this, but California then labeled glyphosate a probable carcinogen and passed a law that would require that the product be labeled as a carcinogen on the product label. If you sell Roundup, you're going have to say "probable carcinogen." Of course, Monsanto was up in arms about that, and they immediately sued the state. So this lawsuit has been going on, but I heard very recently, I think just the last couple of days, that California won the lawsuit. So at the moment, the law still stands. I don't know if Monsanto will take it to a higher court level, but that's very encouraging.

✳ ✳ ✳

I am very happy that Stephanie was able to take all her research and explain it in terms that we could understand. Many times, you know that a chemical is not good for you, but lack the understanding of exactly why and how it harms us. One of the biggest complaints that I hear over and over is how expensive organic food is compared to non-organic. I would never deny that this isn't true and a huge hurdle for many families. But think about how expensive cancer and other diseases are from treatment expenses, loss of wages and possibly loss of life. Many nutritionists have discovered ways to work around the cost issue. You will read about this in greater detail throughout the "My Kitchen" chapter in Part 3. Certainly, one step would be to take all processed food out of your overall diet, which as Stephanie points out is filled with glyphosate-containing sugars from GMO corn and sugar beets. These foods can also be expensive and definitely wreak havoc on your entire system as they contain some of the worst chemicals and preservatives that disrupt your body's own natural metabolic processes.

Food is definitely one of the easiest ways to control the amount of glypho-sate that enters your body. You can do your research and try to buy locally from a CSA (Community Supported Agriculture) where the farmer does not use glyphosate as well as save money. Growing your own food may be prohibi-tive for people who live in the city, but may be an option for others. Vaccines is another area where you can limit the amount of glyphosate by deciding how many and which ones, if any, you should take. Choosing not to live near farms that spray glyphosate may take some investigation, but you can certainly choose whether to place it on your own lawn. You may not be able to prevent contact with it in a park or other outside areas such as a school. However, you can take proactive steps such as by inquiring with the school what type of pesticide management they utilize and asking if they would mind giving you their schedule. I was very friendly when I called the Parks Department in the city I live in, which happens to spray enormous amounts of this toxin. I spoke with a supervisor and explained that I have a very sick child and need to know where and when they are spraying glyphosate, so I can keep him indoors to protect him. He first gave me the whole song and dance about how it is non-toxic, but then was happy to point out that the schedule can be seen online at their website. Another easy thing would be to not directly let your skin come into contact with the grass in a park by siting on it or walking without shoes and socks.

I know a lot of people have a hard time imagining how something that can't be seen with the naked eye can be so toxic. It is no different from when you break a mercury-containing thermometer or light bulb that you can get acutely poisoned, or in the case of glyphosate, it can build up over time. If you want to have a healthy baby that is free of chronic illness then you will have to be thoughtful of all the areas where you can prevent a toxic build up. Remember the principle of the total load theory is that it only takes one last assault to break the camel's back or push you over the edge of the cliff. Use the visual that once you are over the cliff, think how hard it is to climb back up a steep one. This is exactly what I have been experiencing with my son for the past ten years, which is why I never begrudge any of the inconvenient things I do each day to protect my daughter and try to regain my son's health

CHAPTER SUMMARY

Glyphosate is the main chemical ingredient in the widely used pesticide Roundup, which is used to kill weeds, especially on GMO crops. It is also sprayed on non-GMO food crops, such as wheat, sugar cane, and peas, right before harvest as a desiccant (a drying agent).

Some scientists believe that glyphosate replaces the naturally occurring glycine in our body during protein synthesis. A process called molecular mimicry creates a lot of problems in our body, when a glyphosate-contaminated foreign protein resembles a human protein and causes autoimmune disease.

Recently, vaccines have been tested, and some have been found to be contaminated with glyphosate.

Glyphosate disrupts DNA repair, which makes a person more prone to getting cancer.

Another issue is that glyphosate chelates important minerals, causing a deficiency in certain people. It also disrupts the transport system that brings minerals to certain places in the body that they need to go to.

Glyphosate tends to destroy good bacteria in the gut, which can lead to an overgrowth of bad bacteria, further imbalancing the gut flora.

The gut microbes can be disrupted by glyphosate causing them not to be able to produce vital vitamins, nutrients, and other molecules that our bodies need.

Glyphosate may deplete methionine, which is needed for the methylation pathway and sulfation pathway that help our body detoxify itself.

Studies have found high levels of glyphosate in human breast milk, and it is probably being passed from mother to child in utero.

PART 3

Chapter 12

OTHER PARENTS' STORIES
With Corinne Simpson Brown, Katie Wright, and Maria Rickert Hong

I wanted to share some heartfelt stories from other mothers about their children. And it is very important to me that you hear from these moms in their own words. The stories you are about to hear will vary in topic, however they have one common thread that strings them all together. This thread is made up of undying passion, determination, truth seeking, and love that transcends all barriers. Each of these mothers will stop at nothing, no matter how inconvenient, to protect their child and keep them healthy, or to recover their health after an injury. I have something in common with each one of these inspiring ladies, since I too have experienced that same journey each of them has been through. One is a story of prevention, vaccine injury and recovery of health before an autism diagnosis. I am not able to thank them enough for their willingness to share their children's intimate stories for you to learn from. These are some of the most beautiful, intelligent and impassioned women you will ever meet.

The first story is about a lovely family, living on Long Island, that has a beautiful son named Patrick who was diagnosed on the autism spectrum. I first met his mom Corinne when I raffled off a TAGA bike, which is a bicycle that has a stroller attached to it. My husband had bought it for me as a push present, and my daughter had just grown out of it. So I thought it would be great to give it to another family that has a child with autism. Corinne was one of the first people to answer the raffle and win the bike. I knew when I first spoke to her on the phone that there was something so special about her, but it wouldn't be until years later that this would be confirmed when I finally got the chance to meet her in person. Corinne drove all the way out to Sag Harbor so I could interview her for a documentary that I am working on about preventing autism, which is based on this book. We had an extremely intimate interview where she shared many details and deep emotions that were connected to her family's journey. As

I mentioned, they have one child on the spectrum and at the time she already had another baby growing in her belly. She was frightened beyond belief about the health of her unborn child but determined to make sure that this next baby did not suffer the same way as Patrick. Here is her family's story of prevention:

PATRICK'S STORY

Dara: Tell me when was the first time that you noticed something was going on with Patrick?

Corinne: When Patrick was about two months old, he developed very low muscle tone and it was very concerning because I was becoming very afraid to hold him; he was so floppy and he started receiving physical therapy because of his low muscle tone. From that point on I was very concerned about his development, he just seemed very quiet and a little too calm and a little too easy going.

He also had torticollis. What brought it to my attention was he had a little lump behind his ear and I couldn't figure out where it came from. It just appeared one day, so I brought him to the pediatrician and they sent me for a physical therapy evaluation, where they diagnosed him with torticollis—which basically means that he had a weakness on one side of his neck and his neck and his head were favoring one position. He was developing a flat spot on the side of his head and this whole thing was connected to his low muscle tone.

Dara: At what point did you think something was really wrong? You told me about how you started buying books on developmental delays, but you were hiding them and not letting anybody see them. Tell me about that whole period of time, what was going on in your head and what symptoms did you notice that were alarming.

Corinne: I guess he was about nine months old when I came to the realization there was something serious that was hindering his development. He wasn't clapping, he wasn't interested in objects that were not easy for him to grasp, objects that were rolling out of his reach. A lot of it was just a strong mother's intuition. He was very easy, he was very content, he was extremely happy all the time, but he didn't try to do anything. If you're trying to play a game with him, like roll a ball to him and it rolled out of his reach, it didn't matter to him, he was still happy. He wasn't trying to go after it like other babies his age, and while I was taking him to physical therapy, I also noticed that things didn't come naturally to him. He learned how to crawl because she, the physical therapist, showed him how to do it. It wasn't something that he naturally did on his own and I had thought to myself, "God, if he wasn't in physical therapy I wouldn't have known how to teach him to do anything." And being my first child I didn't know that other kids just naturally did these things. Thankfully because he was in physical therapy, Patrick met a lot of his gross motor milestones pretty much on time, but other than that, he was delayed everywhere else.

Dara: Tell me about more of these early signs and the resources you referenced for answers.

Corinne: As we were approaching his first birthday, he was probably about ten months old, I noticed that he wasn't making a lot of babbling sounds, his eye contact had started to disappear, and I noticed he was looking not at me, but over my shoulder a lot. And a couple of times, I noticed that he was laughing and there was nothing that I could see that could have triggered that response. I think during that time I started just looking things up on the internet which I hadn't done before and I had of course that baby book that everybody has, *What to Expect When You're Expecting.* I threw that book out after Patrick's formative years, as there was no way I was going to rely on that book again for any subsequent children.

Dara: My friends and I who have had children with special needs feel it is "The Most Upsetting Book," since every page you turn to tells you all the ways in which your child is behind. Tell us more about your internet research and any resources you had found while searching for answers to Patrick's condition.

Corinne: As he was approaching his first birthday in May, Autism Awareness Month was in the news so the various news organizations were posting the top ten early warning signs for autism, and Patrick was pretty much meeting all of them. Even though he was meeting all these criteria, it still didn't make sense to me. I had just assumed he was delayed. I couldn't even say the word autism, but I think reading different things about the early signs is what led me to start buying books on the subject.

Dara: You told me a story about how you spoke to your husband, and he said, "Oh no, he's got eye contact. He looks at me." Tell me more about this experience.

Corinne: After reading, and starting to become more and more concerned about whether Patrick could possibly have autism, I did mention to my husband that Patrick hadn't been responding to his name. And I remember that he said, "That's not true," and he called his name. After that it was the first time that I remember him actually saying that Patrick was not responding to his name, or I'm pretty sure that he was in the past because it wasn't something I had always worried about but some time around the one-year mark he definitely stopped responding to his name all the time. Sorry [crying].

Dara: No apologies, it's hard, because that type of realization occurs over time. One day you have a moment where you really take stock of what's going on, and you start to compartmentalize a list of all the things that seem a little off, and all of a sudden you have quite a list. So I know exactly what you're talking about when your child stops listening to you. What happens next after you realize that he is no longer responding to his name?

Corinne: Actually, Patrick's physical therapist had asked me if we had his twelve-month doctor's well visit and what their impression was. When I told the physical therapist that Patrick's pediatrician didn't make any major comments, she was very adamant that we take Patrick to a physician who could perform a full evaluation. She wrote down the phone number for me to call and told me that I should have a Special Education evaluation and a speech evaluation, because he wasn't showing any progress. He wasn't clapping, he wasn't pointing, he wasn't developing language or trying to get your attention if he needed something.

Dara: Was it soon after that he finally did get an autism diagnosis, or what occurred next?

Corinne: When he was about thirteen or fourteen months old, they did the whole early intervention evaluation, where he was approved for speech, occupational therapy, feeding therapy, physical therapy, and a special education teacher. At this point, I'm really starting to research autism because now it's obvious that something is not right. He was scoring at a two-month level on almost every measure. After about two months in early intervention, everybody was like, "Once he starts early intervention, you're gonna see such progress, it's so helpful." Nothing helped. He wasn't making any progress at all so I had asked for a recommendation to a developmental pediatrician to have him evaluated for autism, he was eighteen months old at the time. At that point I think in my heart I knew, it wasn't a surprise.

I went in there expecting them to tell me that he had autism, I was hoping that it wasn't going to be that bad, I was hoping he was definitely going to be higher functioning. I don't think she called it autism in that appointment. I think she called it PDD-NOS, which made us feel a lot better. It was the 'nice' way of telling us that our son had autism. That's how we took it.

Dara: I've heard that same story from many parents. Doctors don't normally give that diagnosis of autism before three years of age in case the child "grows out of it." I was told PDD-NOS too. I went home and researched it on the internet and found that PDD-NOS is like an equal sign to autism. So now you have the autism diagnosis and he's obviously getting even more therapy, right? What happens after the diagnosis?

Corinne: Within about two weeks, we had a whole new team of therapists in the house, ABA teachers (I believe Patrick started getting fifteen hours a week of ABA at home in addition to speech), OT, PT, and actually special education, too. Basically, Patrick's day started at 8:30 in the morning, he worked with a therapist until about noon, took a brief nap at noon since he was only eighteen months old, and then they would come back around 2:30, and he'd have another two or three hours of therapy for the day.

Dara: Were you worried at that point that he was not going to get better?

Corinne: Yes. I think my biggest concern was never hearing him speak. It's so difficult because at eight years old, he's still not speaking, so I look back and just feel so bad.

Dara: Let's go back to how you were saying your biggest worry was if he's ever going to speak. Tell me about some other worries of yours. For me, I worry about whether my son is ever going to experience true friendships.

Corinne: I guess my major concern is what's going to happen to him later on in life, after he turns twenty-one? What's going to happen to him then? Where is he going to go, what is he going to do with his life, who will be taking care of him? It seems like it's so far away, but the past eight years have gone so fast that I know that I'm going to turn around and it's going to be here; and we currently don't have a plan in place for him. Years ago I used to worry about building friendships but right now I think because he's not at the point where he's interested in other children, it doesn't upset me, him not having friends. It's not something that he cares about. I know other kids that are higher functioning, they want to be around other kids but they don't know how. He's not even at that point. He doesn't want to be bothered with other kids. For me right now I'm okay with that, for some reason it doesn't upset me.

Dara: Do you or your husband worry about not being around for him?

Corinne: It's, the scariest feeling, because I don't know who's going to take care of him after we're gone. He has two brothers, but that's a huge burden to have to put on them. And who knows what they're going to be like when they get older. Are they going to be able to provide for Patrick? Is it fair to put that on them? I want them to have their lives and not always have to worry about their brother, but what other choice do we have as parents?

Dara: What do you think are some of the things that contributed to Patrick getting autism? Obviously we didn't know the things back then that we know now, but for other parents' benefit, please tell us a little bit about these things so they can learn from us.

Corinne: I did so many things wrong with Patrick. I mean, from the day he was born, he was drinking formula that had horrible chemicals in it. He was drinking out of plastic bottles every single day, I was heating those plastic bottles every single day, and then he was eating processed baby food that I was heating in a microwave. These are some of the little things that all add up in the end. He was toxic from day one, with the processed food I was putting into his body and the fact that he was exposed to so much plastic and radiation.

Dara: Were there any other things that you could think of, like, did you eat differently back then, did you use chemicals in your house or any other things that we now know that we have to stay clear of? I'm trying to get at some of the changes mothers/parents can make to their own health or environment that have remarkable effects on children down the road.

Corinne: Yes. Before he was diagnosed, I didn't know about the chemicals in my house, and the harm they can cause children. I used Lysol, bleach, I even used Dreft laundry detergent. I probably used Johnson's baby shampoo. Everything is so different now that I know what not to put on our bodies and into our bodies.

Dara: Did you recognize anything as what I've been referring to as a trigger, or the straw that broke the proverbial camel's back? For my son, at eighteen months old, he had a vaccination at 6 p.m., and twelve hours later when he woke up in the morning he never spoke again. Most people have regressive autism.

Corinne: I don't have that type of story. Whatever vaccine trigger Patrick had happened very early on. My personal belief was that it was an accumulation of all of these contributing factors, starting when he was two months old and one of his pupils stopped dilating. And looking back, I'm thinking he must have had some type of a stroke related to his vaccines. We had him tested for Horner Syndrome, but everything came back negative. But that was the biggest early clue that something was not right, the fact that one of his pupils was not dilating and nobody could give us any answers on that.

Dara: There is one doctor that had done a lot of research and wrote a book about children having strokes from vaccines and that it's much more common than we think. The symptoms are there with the asymmetry in the face that develops, drooling and loss of function or change in appearance on one side of the face. I believe that strokes are more common among children than people think, especially those that suffer from autism and more specifically vaccine injury.

Now let's talk about the fact that all this is going on in your life. All hell is breaking loose with Patrick, and then you find out you're pregnant. When did you find out you were pregnant with your second child?

Corinne: Patrick was about nine months old when I found out that I was pregnant with my second child.

Dara: Then here you have this child that's falling apart, disintegrating in front of you and you learn you're about to have another child. What's going through your mind?

Corinne: I was petrified, especially once I started thinking that it was autism because I knew that there are a lot of people out there that had multiple children with autism, and that there was a strong possibility that this could happen to my next child. I was so upset over what was going on with Patrick, and to think that I could be doing this all over again, I was completely petrified.

Dara: I totally understand. So your second son, Keiran, is born and you're dealing with Patrick's comprehensive therapy regimen that you mentioned above; what was going through your mind when you looked at this second baby?

Corinne: For Kieran, the first year of his life I was sick, I was a nervous wreck. I lost so much weight, I was just so sick. I couldn't eat, my anxiety and nervousness were out of control. I was constantly looking for signs, to see if there was something not right with Kieran. His eye contact was not great, and of course you know, that's one of the first things you look at so I was so sick for his first year of life, constantly worried and full of anxiety.

Dara: Let's talk about that first doctor's visit. You went with your husband. You guys had a plan. Tell me about the plan.

Corinne: At that point the whole autism diagnosis was new to us. We weren't really sure about anything, about what caused it, where it came from. We decided together as parents that we were going to hold off on vaccinating our son Kieran. So we went to his first doctor's appointment where somehow they convinced us to follow their schedule, and we did end up giving him the first round of vaccines when he was about six weeks old. We went in there as a team, not wanting to give him anything and somehow they made us feel so terrible about wanting to delay the vaccines, that we ultimately did something that we weren't comfortable doing to our son.

Dara: And were you both upset after?

Corinne: Yes. We got home. We look at each other like, "How did we let that happen?" especially because we both felt the same going into the visit, and I think that we just felt so terrible that we let somebody talk us into doing something that we were not comfortable doing, you know, to our child and to think that we did something that could possibly hurt him. We were really upset about it.

Dara: I understand. I remember feeling intense pressure to vaccinate Dylan even though my mommy instinct was telling me not to. Unfortunately, this is very common. And it's unfortunate that many doctors now will threaten not to see your child if you don't follow the vaccination schedule—so it makes it even more difficult.

What happened after that, when you decided that you were not going to do that again?

Corinne: I think after that we felt much better about it and much stronger, especially because we were so devastated that we did it to begin with. Then again, at the same time I think we probably were also putting off doctor's appointments. I didn't want to go to the doctor because I was afraid that they were going to bully me into doing something I didn't want to do.

Dara: That's a terrible feeling. I also stopped bringing Dylan to regular doctors. I only felt comfortable with his functional medicine doctors, since they really understood his health conditions.

So, then, what other things did you do differently? Of course, changing vaccination schedules is a big one, but I'm imagining there are probably other decisions you made with Kieran different than with Patrick, because new information was coming to light and you wanted to take action in trying to prevent a similar diagnosis in Kieran.

Corinne: We immediately started taking Kieran to a chiropractor and from day one we started giving him vitamin D, probiotics, and fish oil. We also avoided fluoride vitamins that his doctor prescribed when Kieran was an infant. We changed all of our household cleaners, everything, to natural cleaning products. Everything in our house was changing over, getting rid of all types of toxic chemicals in our home. I didn't breastfeed any of my kids, I was too afraid.

Dara: Were you scared to give toxins through breast milk?

Corinne: With Kieran I was afraid that I was toxic. The only thing, he was still formula-fed, and we started buying organic formula. We did not heat up plastic any longer. With Patrick, I used that awful bottle warmer most people use, but not with Kieran.

Dara: I did that too with Dylan. I am horrified now when I think that the BPA was just melting into the formula.

Corinne: With Kieran I stuck it in a cup of hot water.

Dara: I used the same exact technique with my daughter. If the bottle was cold, then I would place it in warm water for five minutes to get the chill out. I even carried a Thermos with me that had warm water in it for when I was running errands.

Let's switch to Finn, so you get pregnant a third time, how long after Kieran was Finn born?

Corinne: Kieran was about two and a half years old when I became pregnant for the third time, and thankfully by that time I was completely aware, I didn't put anything bad in my body. Looking back with Patrick I was on antibiotics twice, I took Tylenol frequently. I was taking allergy medication. I don't think I did any of that with

Kieran, I knew better. With Finn, my food was much better, and our house was clean. You know, everything that I ate with Kieran and Finn was natural or organic and no medications. I had always suffered from allergies and I used to take allergy medicine every single day, so the whole time I was pregnant with Patrick I was taking allergy medicine.

Dara: Did the doctor tell you it was safe to take the allergy medicine when you were pregnant with Patrick?

Corinne: I did ask. He just said that there wasn't anything that showed that it was not safe.

Dara: How are your other boys with Patrick's disability? How is that for them?

Corinne: It's affected Kieran, who is sixteen months younger than Patrick, a lot. He's had to grow up a lot quicker, but he is amazing to his brother. He could tell anybody anything about autism. He looks out for him constantly. He tries to take care of him. He does anything to try and help him.

Dara: How is Patrick able to communicate with you right now?

Corinne: He communicates in a couple of different ways. Patrick is extremely connected so he has a really great way of communicating with his eyes if that makes any sense, but he can speak to you by looking at you. He does have some verbal approximations, and he'll take me to things that he wants. He tries any way to get his point across. If all else fails, he'll use a communication device. He uses the communication device to speak for him and he'll be able to tell me what it is that he wants.

Dara: What advice would you give to a friend who is pregnant for the first time?

Corinne: I would tell them to do their own research. I would tell them to rigorously research your doctors and the ingredients that you're going to be putting into your body. Spend the same amount of time as you would research what you're putting into your child's body as you would on buying a car seat or a high chair. I feel like for a lot of new moms, they are so concerned about getting the right car seat and the right high chair, but they're not stopping to look at what are they actually putting into their child's bodies at such a young age. That's something I wish I would've thought of when I was a first-time mom, not worried about having the best car seat and high chair and stroller. But I trusted my doctors to do all of the other stuff for me and I didn't look into anything. I went to the doctor, did what they told me to do, and trusted them instead of listening to my own gut and mother's instinct in being really concerned about what I was putting into my child's body.

Dara: How have your feelings changed towards doctors now?

Corinne: I've lost a lot of faith in the mainstream medical doctors. I just assumed the doctor would want to do what's best for you, not what they're being told to do by I'm assuming pharmaceutical representatives. People with vested interests selling doctors their products is what concerns me the most. I feel that doctors are selling a product instead of really trying to take care of you and keep you healthy.

Dara: If you could look back at Patrick's life, if you could take back anything you did to him, is there anything that you wish you didn't do?

Corinne: I wish that I never vaccinated him, especially looking back, I mean, he was eight pounds. The amount of toxic chemicals that I put into his body, over and over again, for his first year of life. I never read any of the ingredients until after he was vaccinated, and had I known I would never have done that to him.

Dara: Let's talk a little bit about how autism has affected your marriage. You know that the divorce rate amongst special needs families is seventy-five to ninety percent. It's obviously very different.

Corinne: It puts a huge strain on our marriage. I mean we're not fun, we can't relax, we can't just go on vacation. Luckily we both love our son more than anything. And we're totally in this together, but we don't have the same life that we thought we would have. Thankfully we love each other.

Dara: How's Patrick doing now?

Corinne: Patrick is happy. For the most part, he's very happy. He's silly. He's funny. His favorite thing in the world is Mickey Mouse. He is overall a happy kid. The past couple of years he's become a little bit more difficult because he's frustrated, as I mentioned to you earlier. He's very connected and very much aware of his environment, but he can't effectively communicate so he gets very angry and his moods change quite a bit, where he can be very happy and then he gets over stimulated and overwhelmed. Then he can be very upset, but he loves his family. That I do know: that he loves us.

Dara: Does he have any behaviors or symptoms like I was telling you with my son, who has these tics and OCD? Are there any things that someone would notice right away if they hung out with him for a great deal of time?

Corinne: Patrick has a lot of self-stimulatory behaviors, so he's constantly either walking back and forth or jumping up and down. He's calmed down a little bit with that, but he also has exhibited some new behaviors in the past couple of years where if he becomes extremely frustrated, he bites himself, so his hands and wrists are covered in bite marks. The first thing he does when he gets angry or upset is to bite himself and scream. So that's really, really difficult for us because it's so upsetting to watch, and it makes it difficult to go anywhere with him. It happens so much, and we don't know when it's going to happen.

Dara: Do you feel like people around you understand what autism really is? Like you hear a lot about people lose a lot of friends after an autism diagnosis. I cut a ton of people out that I felt weren't sensitive enough. Tell me a little bit about what went on with your friendships.

Corinne: I have a new group of friends that basically all have children in the same situation. You don't relate to your old friends as much as you used to and it's hard. It's really hard. I'm sure they want to understand but at the same time when you're not living it, you see stuff on TV or you read stuff and I don't think they realize how bad it really is or what goes on on a daily basis. I'm sure they sympathize but you don't have the same type of connection that you once did, and your life changes so much. Your focus is so much on your child that you just don't have time for typical friendships anymore.

Dara: Tell me about what your hope is of how things might change and your feelings on not calling it an epidemic. Explain how you feel.

Corinne: I think one of the scariest things is that people are afraid to talk about it. Until people start really acknowledging what the problem is here, I'm afraid, I just don't know how many more kids have to be diagnosed for people to start realizing what a problem it is, but on the other hand I'm afraid that it's starting to become so normal. Everybody has a child now with autism or has a cousin or their next-door neighbor. I am afraid that this new generation isn't going to remember what it was like for our generation where nobody had autism. I think that's something that really scares me.

I felt that Corinne's story was really important to share, so that you would get another perspective on what it's like to try to prevent autism. We all look back in retrospect and wish we had done some things differently, but remember that you can only base your decisions on the information you had at the time. So, please don't beat yourself up about anything that you read and now see that was obvious not to do. My list is endless I promise you that! I have had no choice but to let go of the "what ifs" and forgive myself, although that isn't to say I still don't have my moments. Last night, I had a difficult time falling asleep and allowed myself to think about how sad it is what Dylan has had to endure. I shed some tears for his lost childhood, his ample potential and everything I did not get to watch him experience and still don't. Today is a new day and I sit down to share other people's stories so that my son's journey and their children's experiences may help your child one day.

CHRISTIAN'S STORY

This next story hits very close to home as I have gone through so many of the experiences that Katie echoes, including the tumultuous feelings that go with a child's vaccine injury. It is both my honor and privilege to be given permission to tell the heartbreaking journey about a very special boy. I laid eyes on Christian for the first time when his mother, Katie Wright, appeared on national TV to talk about how her son was catapulted into autism following a vaccine injury. I wish that I could tell you that his story is unique in some way. Unfortunately, I have met too many parents over the years who have experienced the same exact thing, myself included. It's important that you hear the terrifying ordeal that her entire family has been through, and how Christian still suffers today.

I remember sitting in my living room with my husband when the video of what Christian was like before the vaccine injury played on my TV screen. He was bright, sociable, and very alert, not to mention incredibly handsome. Christian spoke in sentences and even was potty-trained at such a young age. You would have thought he was the picture of perfect health. And in the blink of an eye, that all changed. Please hear her story so we can all honor Christian that he did not go through this in vain. I want to share his journey in the hopes that it may inspire some of you to press on to do more research and make a decision that is based on having all the information.

Dara: Tell me how you and Andreas were feeling about the pregnancy.

Katie: Well, I was very healthy. I had no problems conceiving. We were excited. I was thirty-one, and I felt great. I worked. I initially had some morning sickness, but nothing unusual. Then it went away. I worked literally until the day he was born. I had a really trouble-free pregnancy.

I wasn't old and I didn't have any vaccines. I remember at one point they offered me the flu shot and I really didn't know anything about it. I just thought it was overkill. I didn't need that, but at that time they were really pushing it.

Dara: Tell me about his birth. Was Christian born healthy?

Katie: The only thing is he didn't turn around, so they did a C-Section when I was almost thirty-eight weeks. The doctor wanted to do it a little early because he was concerned that maybe there was a little bit less amniotic fluid, but it wasn't an emergency. He ended up being born August 31st, and it was obvious that since there was a long holiday weekend coming up, everybody was going to be away and he wanted to perform the procedure before then.

Dara: Then tell me about his first few days. Was he healthy after he was born?

Katie: He was a little jaundiced. Cognitively, he seemed perfect and healthy, but he definitely was a little bit jaundiced. He was six pounds, seven ounces, nothing wrong with him except for a little jaundice.

He started breastfeeding. It was super; no problem. He had a huge appetite, unlike my second son where it was a nightmare. Christian really took to breastfeeding almost exclusively for the first few months.

Dara: What was he like as a baby?

Katie: Cognitively, he was great. He met every single milestone, sometimes exceeded them. He sat up and he smiled on time. He really bonded with Andreas and me, and my mom. I went back to work part-time. He loved his caregiver. My gosh, he started talking on time, like, "Mama, dada, kitty, go." You know, all those words a little bit before he was one. He did have a bad reaction to that horrible DTaP, Hib, and Hep B at two months. It was like an all-day fever and some yelling, but the doctor assured me it was normal, that it was no big deal. Looking back of course, it was a big deal. It seemed like everything except dying was not a big deal.

Dara: Then how did he react to the four and six month ones?

Katie: Much the same at four and six months. Lots of yelling and all day fever, very upset. When I read now that they say, "Well might have sore-ness," it was much worse than that, but he bounced back. He really did bounce back. He was fine, except for after about six months he did start catching more colds. He began with ear infections, and then a few months later eye infections.

Dara: It sounds like even despite these reactions to the two- and four-month vaccines, he developed normally. Is that right?

Katie: Yes. The only thing was actually he was a terrible sleeper. He would nap an hour a day, from when he was two months old, then sleep nine hours a night, tops. I didn't really understand, looking back he was sweating a lot, which is a sign of mercury toxicity. He was sweating a lot, but I really didn't think much of it.

Dara: Did he get mercury vaccines?

Katie: Oh yeah, oh yeah. He was sweating a lot following those vaccines. Christian was really such a bright baby, and so aware, hyper-aware of everything. He has one of those really sensitive brains. He was aware of everything around him. He always had really good hearing and was very curious.

Dara: For some reason as Sid Baker said, those are the ones. For whatever reason, that sensitivity makes them so sensitive to autism.

Katie: Right, exactly, like he always had really good hearing, strong response to texture and food, but in a normal way, in a curious way.

Dara: When did you first start seeing any soft signs that maybe something wasn't right?

Katie: Oh God, after the MMR at twelve months. I noticed in pictures. I look back in the pictures before he was twelve months. He looked right in the camera and smiled or waved to me. You would never guess. It drives me crazy when you realize you've missed the signs. Totally normal. After the MMR—that was a bad one—more screaming and yelling. He just didn't seem to rebound. He seemed more fussy, seemed easily irritated. He started making a little bit of strange hand motions. Looking back, he was beginning to do stimming.

Dara: Now was this his big MMR reaction the really bad one that you talk about?

Katie: Yeah, that was a bad one. We get home, and he screams. He's screaming and screaming. It seems to last forever. The fever is so bad. I called the pediatrician. Again, no big deal. "Give him Tylenol. Give him Tylenol."

The worst possible advice. We give him Tylenol. Still at night time it gets worse. I just wish we had gone to the ER. Our pediatrician was like, "Okay, we'll get him in a bath of ice." I get him in a bath of ice. His temperature comes down, but he's still screaming. He was screaming and awake almost all night and didn't eat anything. He wouldn't breastfeed, nothing. That was awful. Then he seemed better in the morning, but like foggy, a little bit out of it. Then soon after that the diarrhea started.

Dara: How often was that?

Katie: Oh God, like two or three times a day. Then we started noticing horrible rashes on his backside, like really bad. I just thought, "Okay well, this is like an episode of diarrhea and I will put ointment on it." Then I noticed it was like very persistent eczema. Again, I didn't think that much of it because I have eczema and I have psoriasis on my hands sometimes and my elbows. It comes and goes. I later learned that this was another risk factor when a parent has these things. I just kept thinking it would go away. It did wax and wane, but his attention was never quite as sharp afterwards. Then at eighteen months it was another bad reaction, then kind of like a free fall.

Dara: What was the bad reaction to at eighteen months?

Katie: Eighteen months there was the DTaP and I think again like the stupid Hib or the Hep B. That's another thing, it's never one vaccine, which I feel is so misleading in the research. The new Schaeffer Study recently studied the reaction of siblings who got the MMR. However, he measured siblings who got the MMR alone. Now I don't know anybody who got the MMR alone with their first child, with their autistic child. Then he also measured kids who got the MMR until the age of five. I think the fact that our kids are getting the MMR at twelve months versus ten years ago, when they were getting it at age two. It's a big difference.

Dara: Then how did the doctor react to Christian after the twelve-month visit where he had the diarrhea. Did you go back and tell her?

Katie: She was like, "Oh well, it's no big deal." Literally, I could have said anything except death I think, and it would have been no big deal. Even a touch of annoyance frankly—annoyance that I was calling again. When I called about other things she didn't dismiss me, or wasn't condescending, but this, yes totally was to vaccine reactions.

Dara: Then tell me what happened at the eighteen-month visit. You went in, and he wasn't sick or anything?

Katie: No, but he hadn't fully rebounded. He was becoming more sickly like again after twelve months ear infection, eye infection, and I'm pretty sure a coxsackie virus. At eighteen months, he just started to become sicker and definitely less focused; I noticed more stimming, like the kind of weird running in place. I started to notice that after eighteen months, he was more fixated on his hands, but not quite flapping. It started to become more difficult for him to sleep at night, lots more crying. I think it was the beginning of PANDAS. He was extremely clingy with me and had massive separation anxiety. It got so bad, we could only have one babysitter. Also, we would endure hours of screaming.

Dara: What was going on specifically for him developmentally from the eighteen-month to twenty-four-month period?

Katie: He was still walking, talking. He was the king of the playground. He had excellent fine and gross motor skills. He could do everything at the playground; we played hide and seek still. He would say, "Good night mama, see you in the morning." He would say to Andreas, "Daddy loves Christian, right? Mommy loves Christian, right? I love you. See you in the morning. When can I drive the car?" He loved to pretend to drive Andreas's car, sitting on his lap. He would call my mom; he would pretend to talk to her on the phone. Then by twenty-four months it was all gone. I guess between twenty, maybe twenty-two months, he started losing almost all of his language capabilities. He became hysterical if anyone he didn't know approached him.

My mother-in-law had been out of the country for six or seven months. We tried to prepare him that she was coming home. We showed him pictures. When she came he screamed, he wouldn't go near her. She's a very nice woman. Every new person terrified him. I think he just couldn't process it and was really scared. The PANDAS was causing so many problems in his mind. It is my theory that the measles had infected his brain by then and his gut. Then he was diagnosed around twenty-four months, we got the whole spiel about, "Early intervention, will fix it all, you just have to do super intense early intervention." Things got dramatically worse, and I don't blame the therapist. I just think it was ridiculous. I get migraines. It'd be like giving me a behavioral intervention to stop a migraine. How stupid, right? Behavioral interventions to stop menstrual pain?—It's never going to work.

Dara: You know I feel the same way. Now did he have any vaccines at twenty-four months old?

Katie: Thank goodness we didn't. He was supposed to get the flu shot I think around twenty-four months, but he was so sick that I cancelled it, thank goodness. At this point he was sick all time. Around twenty-four months he got a Staph infection from stepping on something. He was in the hospital overnight, then shortly after that he got pneumonia. Then he got Coxsackie again.

Dara: Did he still have diarrhea at this point?

Katie: Yes, bad diarrhea at that point, and then of course antibiotics were given. Then he got cellulitis in both eyes and almost went blind. It was so scary. The eye becomes huge, puffy, and red. We had to put eyedrops in, more antibiotics. It was a cavalcade of sicknesses—and yet still no alarm really from my pediatrician. Then after he was diagnosed, obviously this kept happening. They just didn't connect it and it's absurd that they didn't see these illnesses as warning signs. He was still functional when he was diagnosed. He was still potty training himself. He still had about a dozen words in his vocabulary even after the diagnosis. He still could respond to his name. He still enjoyed being read to after his diagnosis. Then it was just a few months after we started such intense behavioral therapy, we started RDI (relationship development intervention). We also did floor time and speech for the next six months.

For the next six months after his diagnosis he got steadily worse. Everything became worse. Then by . . . let's see . . . twenty-six months, twenty-seven months he had lost every single word. He's never spoken spontaneously again. His bowel problems became much worse, as did the stimming. Around twenty-four to twenty-six months he was waking up at night screaming, just screaming and sleeping maybe two to three hours then going back to sleep. And constant diarrhea, waking up, smearing feces all over his bed, that kind of thing.

Dara: Did you still have the expectation at this point, you and your husband, that he would get through it and get better?

Katie: Yeah, because my parents took us to every specialist, like Boston Children's, and the Presbyterian and Cleveland Clinic. They were all impressed with him. We had a home movie of before the vaccine injury. The thinking was, "Oh if he was like that before, he'll get it all back. It'll be fine." Meanwhile Andreas and I keep pressing, "Well what about him being sick all the time?" They gave me the usual dumb advice like wash his hands a lot, make sure he has a good appetite or whatever. I was feeding him fries, yogurt, and milk, all the stuff he was craving by then. They were not very concerned. Then I remember I had spoke to someone who did the GFCF (Gluten-Free Casein-Free) diet and the doctor at Columbia was like, "That's unscientific, and it's dangerous. Don't do it." They are always obsessed with charlatans and hucksters out there. Meanwhile what they were selling was more hucksterism, like all it takes is behavioral intervention to magically repair severe brain trauma.

Dara: When did you guys put two and two together, that it was the vaccines?

Katie: I wish I could say I was smarter about it. The problem was when he was twenty-four months old, I had had my second son. . . . He had just been born. I was very overwhelmed with that. He was an extremely colicky baby, seemed to be showing much more soft signs of autism than Christian did. Like extremely colicky, he didn't breastfeed. Of course, he got the Hep B shot with the mercury. He was born in 2003. It was legal to still have mercury in all vaccines, as you know, until 2004. I was very preoccupied with him, but then I remember Andreas called me, after Christian was two. He said, "I've been hearing this stuff about mercury and you should definitely not give it to Mattias. Make sure there's no more mercury in his vaccines."

I, of course was like, "Ahh, those people are crazy, of course vaccines are safe. The government says so." At least I did stop Mattias from getting more mercury vaccines, although he continued with the schedule, I think until he was twelve months old, at which point I stopped.

I stopped before the MMR actually. I really didn't want to think about that, because it was so painful. I wouldn't really read much about it, or I avoided it altogether. Then finally, when Christian was about two and a half, I read the Karyn Seroussi book *Unraveling the Mystery of Autism and Pervasive Developmental Disorder*.

Before that the first book on autism I read was *Let Me Hear Your Voice*, by Catherine Maurice, which was basically, "All you need to do is behavioral stuff." In fact, my mom and I tracked Catherine down. We talked to her. She advised that we just do what she did and don't fall for those hucksters. Her kids are healthy. They didn't really have a regression. Anyway, so I really wanted to believe everything would be okay, so I did what she said. Then after I read the Karyn Seroussi book, David Kirby was on Imus. I remember my mom called me and told me to listen. Then I was like, "Oh my God." I bought his book and I read it in a few days; I literally wanted to throw up so many times during the course of reading that book.

Dara: His book, *Evidence of Harm*, speaks about the harmful effects of vaccines. Is this when you put it all together looking back in retrospect?

Katie: I remember talking to a few friends. Some of their children would cry or had fevers, but nothing like Christian had looking back. I don't know why I was so trusting. I was brought up to trust doctors. When I realized the connection between vaccines and these symptoms Christian was exhibiting, I examined his vaccine schedule. For the first time, I really looked at it and compared the dates. It took me so long to recognize that the vaccines had a direct relationship with Christian's emerging symptoms and illnesses.

I looked at the dates and I was like, "Oh my God, that was right after the MMR, oh my God." Then I remember looking at potential side effects, which I'd never looked at before, and I'm like, "Oh my God, he had every single one of those." He had the persistent screaming, the going stiff in my arms, the fever that lasted so long, the refusal to breastfeed the red mark injection site, and then the problems sleeping for a long time. I was like, "Oh my God, he had every single one." He was really a classic regressive kid.

Dara: Did you ever get the doctor's office to admit that he had any reactions to the vaccines?

Katie: This time no. Between when he was eighteen months and two years old we moved from Greenwich to New Canaan. After I read the David Kirby book, I just assumed like every other person from around the time Christian was born in 2001 that the mercury was all out of the vaccines. I assumed, because that's what I'd heard. Then when I read in his book that they were still in—it was voluntary until 2004—I remember feeling nauseous. I called up the old pediatrician's office. I said, "You know, my son has been diagnosed with autism." I asked if I could speak with the doctor. The receptionist asked, "Why?" I said "He's got autism. I want to ask about the vaccines."

I remember the pediatrician didn't want to talk to me, which was weird. She didn't want to talk to me, and I was really annoyed, I'm sure because of the autism issue. Then I wanted to speak with a nurse, and they were very hostile. And then I said something like, "Well I can come to you. I'm going to come to you if you don't talk to me." Then I said, "Can you tell me if any of his vaccines had Thimerosal? I'm sure they didn't, but it would make me feel better if you could tell me." Then she got really defensive, the nurse that is. She's like, "Why are you asking?" I said, "I'd like to know. I have a right to know," fully expecting her to quell my worries. Then she said, "We use what was on the shelf. We weren't going to throw away perfectly good vaccines. It was legal, everything Christian received was perfectly legal until 2004." I think I hung up the phone, and I threw up. I really did throw up that time. I was like, "Oh my God, there was so much mercury."

Dara: Had you gone to a functional medicine doctor by this point?

Katie: Finally after that we went to see Nancy O'Hara, who like a lot of doctors had a long waiting list. It was really hard to find them then, especially in Connecticut. She had a three-month waiting list or something. I guess we saw her before Christian was three. She gave us great advice. She said, "You've got to do the GFCF diet, do it for real." I said, "Okay." I was scared, because he wasn't eating anything, but I did it. She told us in a very professional manner, she's like, "More vaccines for him would be detrimental." I was relieved. I still trusted doctors. I wanted somebody to tell me not to do it. I said, "All my friend's kids got the same vaccine. Why are they fine?"

She's like, "These kids are like a canary in a coal mine. They're just set up to have bad reactions, extreme reactions." Then she referred me to something about how the mercury in these kids stays in their brain, they can't excrete it, which made perfect sense. It wasn't overnight. It was progressively a lot worse over the course of six months. Mercury doesn't cause brain damage in twenty-four hours, but it gets worse and worse. She really tried to help us. He was just so hyper and crazy. The supplements didn't really help at that point.

Dara: He was too sick at that point. What about seizures? Did Christian ever suffer from them?

Katie: He started to have absence seizures, looking back. One doctor that we showed her the video and she said, "I think that's an absence seizure. He seems out of it." It was hard to recognize them, but looking back definitely absence seizures.

DB: Was he still spiraling down at three?

Katie: Spiraling, screaming all the time, really bad attacks of GI pain, he was just miserable. I was afraid to drive anywhere because within a few moments he would start screaming at the top of his lungs and try to break out of his car seat, hitting himself. I had panic attacks because I was dreading having to drive anywhere with him because if I was alone in the car it would be so bad.

Dara: At what point did you think to yourself, "This is not going to get better so easily?"

Katie: Oh, I'm such a die-hard believer, I just kept thinking, "I can get him back. I can get him back." I felt such an enormous responsibility like thinking, "I'm a failure. My life has no meaning. I've ruined my son's life unless I can get him back." Then we moved because I thought part of the problem was he wasn't getting a good ABA and speech therapist, so we moved to New York. I thought that was the problem. Then when he was four we finally found Dr. Krigsman who really helped with the diarrhea. He was tremendously helpful with the diarrhea. That gave me a lot of hope. All these things helped physically, but nothing helped his brain deterioration.

Dara: So Christian was two when Mattias born. You also mentioned he was showing more soft signs?

Katie: Yes, definitely. Super touchy. Horrible eater. Horrible sleeper. Crying all the time.

Dara: Were you nervous that the same thing was going to happen to him that happened to Christian?

Katie: Oh yeah, I was terrified. I was so afraid.

Dara: When did you finally feel safe—that it wasn't happening to him?

Katie: Until he was six months it was awful, but honestly I had to give up caring for him. We had to hire a full-time nanny to care for him because I was literally with Christian every second of the day, trying to work with him and doing floor time. Taking him places, going to school with him and going to sports with him. I regret that so much. It's so sad how I, really I just had to give up Mattias's babyhood. I was very grateful I did find this wonderful nanny who loved him like her own child. The first six months of his life I didn't go anywhere with him alone, probably not for a year because I was always with Christian. He was so sick and at that point Christian couldn't be with anyone but me or his father.

Dara: When this is happening what are families and friends around you thinking and how are they reacting? Did you feel they were supportive?

Katie: Yeah, I think in the beginning people are really supportive because it was easier for them, because they saw his regression. Everybody realized it was so dramatic. They were really concerned. Nobody had ever seen something like that before where a two-year-old loses every word of their vocabulary, the horrible stimming, the fecal smearing. They were all thinking like, "Okay we're going to get this under control. Now we've figured out what's wrong, it's going to be fine." My mom went with me to all these doctors. We were certain at first that it was going to be fine. As the years go on, people become less interested for sure and less supportive, just impatient. They just give up and they just don't want to hear about it anymore.

Dara: Do you find that you lost friends over the years?

Katie: Totally, yeah. I lost almost all my friends. I made new friends thankfully, but all my new friends have kids on the spectrum.

While my other friends were talking about getting into preschools and all that, Christian wasn't doing any of that. I didn't have the time and I didn't have the interest to hang around with my old friends. At first they were really supportive, then after a time I could tell they were horrified, not in a way like, "Oh that's gross" but like, "Oh my God, what's happening." It was also very painful for me because a friend of mine in particular I used to do everything with, her son was the same age. It was just too painful. It was just going to her house would remind me of the things Christian used to be able to do, like play in the backyard. I just couldn't be there anymore. It was just too painful.

Dara: Once he stopped getting sicker and his speech didn't return and you're obviously doing so many things with functional medicine doctors—what are you and Andreas thinking at this point?

Katie: You know, I think what helped me was to dig deeper into the research and go to Autism Research Institute Conferences. That really helped me. For Andreas that didn't help, he didn't want to do that. He just wanted to focus on Christian day-to-day, think about what was working and what wasn't. He kept very detailed logs of his daily activities. We really lived day-to-day. Of course we agree, there will be no more vaccines. We didn't want to think about the future or talk about it for many years.

Dara: How was Christian letting you know he was in pain?

Katie: Laying on tables and chairs all the time to put pressure on his stomach. Looking back I'm sure he had bad headaches with the sudden onset of screaming. Before Dr. Krigsman it was like big undigested food coming out as number two, then after his treatment it was a lot better, but it was still happening. Lots of screaming. He didn't sleep through the night for three years, until he was five probably. We'd go someplace—we'd have to leave after five minutes.

Dara: You decided to stop vaccinating his brother at the twelve-month mark?

Katie: Yes. He totally rebounded and became healthy. He blossomed. He developed tons of words. He became—most importantly—really social. As he became very social, I exhaled because I thought, "Oh this is great." Christian had never sustained that like this. Mattias was really interested in other kids and sought them out, then I really felt, "Oh thank God."

Dara: It seems like Christian could have saved his life?

Katie: Yes, oh for sure. If I had kept vaccinating my second son, without a doubt. He'd be autistic for sure, especially if he had gotten the MMR.

Dara: Then tell me what Christian is like today. I know with my son, even though he's not neurotypical, he still has such a personality. We love him for that. You know what I mean? Tell me about Christian.

Katie: I love Christian so much, but he is still profoundly affected. He has been a pretty consistent non-responder. He developed severe epilepsy last year and he was having full and grand mal seizures. Our life became a lot more complicated, because I could never leave him alone, whereas before he could take a shower and I could be in the other room putting away laundry or something. Now I have to sit there because he's had seizures in the shower and it's just become harder to do things. Actually our life is harder than it was for a long time because of the epilepsy. We did three different EEGs. They always show nothing, which is almost typical for him, for kids like him.

Now that he's in puberty he has severe hypoglycemia. A couple times a month he will try to strike himself so hard, it'll be like an emergency. I'll need someone to come home and help me. His bus driver just asked me to get him a helmet for the bus. It's just awful. It's still awful. I do feel like his personality is better. He's more there, he can be so sweet and he hugs me. He just loves his family so much. In a way he used to be just so out of it all the time. He's not like that anymore.

Dara: Do you feel like he's a happy child?

Katie: Like fifty percent of the time he's happy. The other fifty percent he's struggling still with GI pain and the parasites. He was miserable, just miserable from ages two to five. Miserable one-hundred percent of the time, so it's better now. It used to be better, then it got worse, after the seizures.

Dara: How is that to watch your child go through an experience like this?

Katie: Horrible. It looks like he's going to die. It is so terrifying. It's rare things are as bad, as dramatic as you see in a movie, but this is so dramatic and awful. It makes me furious, I get incensed with rage that this is happening to him.

Dara: Do you ever get fearful of the seizures?

Katie: Yes, it's the number one cause of premature deaths. Oh God, last Christmas we were walking on a pier, I was holding his hand. He had a grand mal seizure and just fell into the ocean. We had to swim to go rescue him in the ocean and flag down another boat.

Dara: Tell me a little bit about what you would like parents to learn from your story that we discussed today?

Katie: Crying and screaming is a bad vaccine reaction; to listen to your gut and just stop. I would not vaccinate at all until your child is three. If you must, I'd do one at a time and pay such close attention; and don't give Tylenol, which only aggravates it.

Dara: Then from everything you've learned—which I know is so immense, because you're so much an integral part of the autism community— what do you wish you knew then, that you know now, not for you to feel guilty? Because, I've got thirty things that I wish I did different, but more for parents who are reading this book, and they're not sure how important each of the things that the doctor talks about. What would you tell them?

Katie: If your kid has GI problems, do the Specific Carbohydrate Diet right away. Don't let yourself be talked into the whole "It's dangerous" crap. I think though it's great that the gluten issue has become a lot more prevalent in the media. Even though the medical community is dragging their heels, you see consumers going gluten free because it just helps them. It's not a fun thing, I'm not doing it because it's trendy like doctors seem to believe. If your child is sick a lot, think about PANDAS and most importantly if you live in Connecticut or Mass. if you experience like your child has these regressive symptoms get the Lyme test, but get the western blot only. The other one, the cheaper one is fifty percent false negative.

Dara: Do you think that autism is at epidemic levels?

Katie: Yes, one-hundred percent.

Dara: Why do you think they have trouble acknowledging it; mainstream medical professionals aren't calling autism an epidemic?

Katie: Money. Oh I think to do that, they all know what's causing it, and they're terrified and money. Because, if the vaccines are causing it, so many people are in so much trouble at the CDC and NIH. Their whole careers are at stake. Parents of young kids don't want to hear it, because they don't want to believe this, because it's so scary. Pharma owns CDC. It's a revolving door.

Dara: Okay. Do you think autism can be prevented?

Katie: One-hundred percent. Listen, maybe there actually are some rare cases where I do think it's genetic, but let's say ninety-five percent aren't. I do know of a woman who didn't vaccinate and her kid just has autism, and also turns out that her brother has autism. I'm sure there are rare cases.

Dara: I can't thank you enough Katie for sharing your difficult experiences with our readers.

Katie: Please! I'm real happy you're doing this. I can't wait to read it. It'll be a great resource.

✳ ✳ ✳

Hearing those words above from Katie makes all my hard work worth it. This book may have been written over a period of about one year, but just like Katie I have been on a long journey with my son for about a decade.

I know Christian's story was probably pretty hard to read at times, but please imagine how difficult it must have been for Katie to relive every detail for all of you. My admiration and respect for Katie's family and what they have had to endure is immense. I can meet a mother of a child with autism for the first time knowing nothing about her and she already commands much of my respect just for what she goes through each day. Nobody knows better what she goes through than another parent of a child with autism.

Katie's son's vaccine-induced autism or injury may seem so extreme to those of you reading about it, but unfortunately I know too many families to count that have shared the same exact experience. It is a shame that we do not have a good reporting system that actually gets used. Parents don't know how to report a vaccine reaction and doctors are not urging them to either.

My heart bleeds every time I see another child like Dylan, Patrick, and Christian when I am just out and about doing my errands or looking on Facebook. I just want to scream at how many children are affected and then round them all up to try to help them. For this reason, I am in the process of getting my health coach certification from the Institute of Integrative Nutrition to help as many of them as I can.

So all I ask is that you honor Christian's story by doing the research, getting all the facts, and making sure your child does not possess one or more risk factors that would make them more susceptible to a vaccine reaction.

RYAN'S STORY

The final story you are about to hear is one of great importance, since it ultimately describes almost every child before they get a chronic childhood illness or descend into the abyss of autism. In this interview, Maria describes all the details of how her children were displaying what we in functional medicine call soft signs that something is amiss with a child's immune system. The symptoms will vary from child to child. However, the fact remains the same that their bodies' physiology is getting off kilter, and without intervention nobody can tell you how deep the damage might go. As you have read throughout this book, the reasons each child's immune system falters are unique to every child.

If you only learn one thing from my book, I hope you take away that it is much more difficult to fix a body once illness has taken over than it is to prevent it from happening in the first place. But the next best thing is to learn how to notice the soft signs and stop illness in its tracks before the effects become devastating, as in the case of my son's autism.

Maria's children, like my own daughter, Jessica, are extremely lucky that their mother is very intelligent and had an "aha" moment in which she was able to put two and two together and figure out that the daily choices she was making were contributing to her child's illness. Please remember that nobody is to blame, including yourself for your child's illness. How could you possibly know information that was not presented to you at the time? I commend you for the mere fact that you have picked up this book and have been open to information that is outside the realm of mainstream thinking. I hope you continue your journey of information seeking, since there are so many more amazing books on this very subject—including the one Maria wrote.

I first met Maria through a documentary film project that I got involved with called "Documenting Hope." The film's goal is to show how children with chronic illness can get better and how some even fully recover through diet and other holistic interventions. I did not know much about Maria's personal story until I purchased her book, *Almost Autism*, which came out last year. It was after reading her story that I realized we had much in common. We both had a child who was quite ill and our second one was showing many of the soft signs that we addressed, and in turn we were able to prevent a childhood chronic illness from occurring in the sibling. Maria is also a certified health coach so you will notice that I ask her questions that pertain to her personal story, as well as the people she treats.

Dara: The first question I ask everybody is do you think autism is increasing?

Maria: Yes. Absolutely, I remember when I was pregnant with my first son, I think the autism rate was about 1 in 166. I think they now officially say that it's 1 in 68, although the previous year they had said that it was 1 in 50.

Dara: Do you think there is an epidemic of autism and other child chronic illnesses?

Maria: Yes. If you talk to any elementary school teacher or nurse, or just any grandparent that has been around kids for a while, they'll tell you that kids today are not the same as kids used to be. When I was growing up, I only knew of one child with any kind of chronic condition, that was one boy who had asthma. Now when you go into the nurse's office at school, you see a whole wall full of EpiPens and inhalers. You see classrooms that are nut-free, and the cafeterias are required to be nut-free as well. So aside from autism, you see definite increases in things like asthma and food allergies, especially anaphylactic allergies, not just to peanuts but to dairy and all sorts of unusual things. That certainly didn't happen when I was a kid.

You can also talk to elementary school teachers and you can find out that kids these days don't have the fine motor skills that they used to. In fact, I think that's one of the reasons why they're getting rid of cursive writing, because kids just can't do it these days. Its little hints and little nudges all over the place that tell us that our kids just aren't healthy these days.

Dara: That's a pretty big hint that nobody can do cursive.

Maria: I know. Just a few kids these days.

Dara: You talk in your book titled *Almost Autism* about your child almost having autism. Can you tell us about this concept of "almost autism?"

Maria: Oh yeah. When I was trying to figure out what was going on with my older son with all the symptoms that he had, when I would research them I would find autism. To me, he did not have autism, but there was a lot of overlap between what was going on with him and with kids that did have autism. In fact, when I finally realized that he did have sensory processing disorder, and I read Dr. Kenneth Bock's book, *Healing the New Childhood Disorders*, where he talks about allergies, asthma, ADHD, and autism being on the same spectrum, I'm like, "That's it! That makes sense!" He pieced it all together for everybody, that it's really what's going on underneath is what we should be looking at, instead of just the label. I think a lot of people get hung up on the label of autism or PDD-NOS; I think if I had pushed hard enough for a diagnosis I could have gotten that for my son. I certainly see sensory processing disorder as being on that spectrum.

Dara: You have two children. Can you tell us if they were both affected by chronic illness and was one more than the other?

Maria: They were both affected, my older one far more so than my younger one. My younger one had minor issues, but I was able to catch them and understand what was going on with him, because I had already been through it all with my older son.

Dara: Let's go back to when your older child was born. Was he healthy at birth?

Maria: He was healthy, although he did have a traumatic birth experience. Other than that, yes he was healthy up until three months of age. In fact, I was looking at pictures a couple years ago and I realized just how healthy he was at that age, at three months, because you could stand him up against an ottoman and he would actually stand. He could sit up supported, which indicates that he had very strong muscles and strong core muscles. Then you fast forward a couple months, and he's had an ear infection, antibiotics, really bad colic, and projectile vomiting. Then, at six months, he could not sit up supported. At eight months, he could only crawl backwards.

    Then he finally began to crawl again, what's called army crawling on the ground. He did that until he was 19 months old. He did not walk until he was 20 months old. That period from about three months until 20 months was lengthened because he had developed very low muscle tone, when in fact he had not had that before. He had actually had very strong muscle tone and we have pictures to prove that.

Dara: What is army crawl?

Maria: Army crawl is when a baby is down on the floor crawling with its elbows, that's as opposed to what's called cross crawl or creeping, which is when the baby is on the hands and knees, which is what you want for a baby. My son only cross-crawled for three weeks before he walked, that's not good, because it's that cross crawling that actually integrates a lot of those primitive reflexes. In fact, if your baby does not cross crawl, it means that a lot of those primitive reflexes will be retained and that they can have all sorts of problems later on with their vision, hearing, coordination, and posture.

    Even if a baby doesn't army crawl, a lot of other problems that can be seen with crawling are butt scooting or dragging a leg behind it as it crawls. That's a sign of a developmental delay or neurodevelopmental damage. I wish that pediatricians would read this book and not just blow off that it's just a different style of moving around or a different style of locomotion and all babies are different. So if a baby is army crawling, it means that he doesn't have enough muscle tone to be able to pick himself up on his hands and his knees to move around. It has a lot to do with his core muscle strength, too. You'll find, if you have a child with autism or ADHD or a neurodevelopmental disorder, that typically a lot of them do not have core muscle strength. Because of that, they don't have good gross motor control. And because of that, they don't have good fine motor skills either. It's all just domino effect, one thing after another. Army crawling, especially for a long period of time, is a huge indicator that your child has neurodevelopmental damage. As a parent, you have got to really pay attention to that and really push for your child.

Dara: Let's go back. Martha Herbert talks a lot about stress: environmental stress, physical stressand psychological stress. He had a traumatic birth, as you said. Do you think, looking back, that stress may have contributed to him developing an illness?

Maria: Yeah, absolutely. A traumatic stress event during birth is one of the potential causes for what's going on with kids with developmental delays or neurodevelopmental disorders, it's one of the recognized causes. In fact, even before he was born, I was working on Wall Street. I was an equity research analyst at a sell-side investment bank. That's a very stressful job—I worked from 7 a.m. to 7 p.m., that was a regular day. Things happen on the stock market. You've got to be able to analyze it very quickly, because people want to make money on it right away, so that's very stressful. When Dr. Herbert talks about stress, stress during pregnancy certainly played a part, as well as stress during childbirth too.

Dara: I had my own share of stress during pregnancy, being on bed rest, and being so worried about Dylan. I had a traumatic birth, as well. I think it's unfortunately very common to have that happen. Maureen McDonnell, is a nurse who helped plan some of the Autism Research Institute Conferences. She talks a lot about how important it is to really lay out a birth plan and have your doctor sign it. So unless there's an emergency, we're sticking to this, and it's something you can bring with you to the hospital, in case another doctor from the practice is there.

Maria: If I were to have another child, I probably would not even go to a hospital, honestly. I hold my own webinars every month in my health coaching practice. I interviewed Jennifer Margulis who wrote *The Business of Baby*. It's now called *Your Baby Your Way*. After I read her book and I interviewed her, I would have done everything completely differently. I would have had my baby either at home or in a midwifery center. I definitely would have had a midwife. I would have not let them clamp the cord as soon as the baby is born, because the baby needs that cord and the nutrients in there from the placenta to help it thrive. Research has shown that early cord clamping is related to things like ADHD and neurodevelopmental disorder. There's so much I would have done differently, too. If you look at the US, we actually have, I believe, one of the highest cesarean rates in the world. I believe it's around thirty percent.

Dara: It is thirty percent. You're correct.

Maria: I don't think a lot of it is necessary. I think a lot of it is because it's more convenient for the doctor and/or for the mom. They don't realize the health risks of having a child born via cesarean that your child is more likely to have asthma, allergies, autism, or a neurodevelopmental disorder because of that. A large part of that is because they don't pick up the good gut flora that comes from going through the mother's vaginal canal. That's the number one reason. If you don't do that, then the baby is picking up whatever germs are just lying around in the hospital.

Dara: That is something we talk extensively about in this book, inoculating the baby with the vaginal secretions when you have to have a C-section. We definitely drive that point home.

Maria: Then the other part that probably doesn't get talked about as much is that the vaginal contractions that the baby works against as it's pushing through the vaginal canal actually help to prime the nervous system and the neurodevelopmental system of this child. It has a large part to play with retained reflexes. A lot of these kids who are born by cesarean have a lot of retained reflexes, which is really interesting too. That's kind of under-discussed.

Dara: That's very interesting. Let's go back to what you noticed at three months. You're starting to see these changes. Did anything specific happen at three months?

Maria: I looked back at the record, and he did get seven vaccinations on one day. Shortly thereafter, he developed this oozing out of his eye. I was like, "What is this?" I took him back to the doctor. It turned out he had an ear infection, which he wasn't screaming or anything from, but it was just this weird oozing out of his eye. They gave him antibiotics. It's really hard to piece it together, as a mom, day by day, years later, because you can't remember exactly the course of events that happened.

I do know that he was healthy and very strong at three months, and then this slow slide downwards into a state of being unhealthy, and in fact, where his muscle tone was so low that he was a floppy baby. People would comment that he was like a little Raggedy Andy doll. He was just like a little floppy sack of potatoes. He had no muscle tone anymore. It didn't dawn on me that he shouldn't have been that way, because he was my first child. Any time I brought anything up to the doctors, they're like, "Don't worry about it. Kids develop differently. You're just a nervous first-time mother. You don't know what you're talking about."

Dara: That's a very common, unfortunate thing that we keep hearing over and over from parents, including myself. I brought Dylan into the doctor and said he's no longer speaking. She told me, "Oh, New Yorkers are crazy. He'll talk soon."

Maria: Exactly. I was living in New York City, too, as well.

Dara: That's unfortunate. I'm glad you mentioned that. When did you first really say to yourself, "Okay. That's great that the doctor said that he's developing fine, but no. He's not fine." What happened to really make you have to seek an answer for him?

Maria: We had red flags all along the way. Unfortunately those doctors did push back against them. It wasn't until he entered preschool at age three. He was highly verbal at home and he would chat nonstop. At preschool he didn't talk. In fact, they wondered if he did have autism, because he was nonverbal at school.

It was that there was this thunderstorm that happened when he was at school one day. He flipped out, because it got really dark. He got really upset, and he thought that it was nighttime and that I had not come to pick him up. And he just flipped out. It was just such an extreme reaction. I'm like, "Okay. This is it. This is enough. I'm tired of being told that I'm crazy, that there's nothing wrong with my child. There is something wrong. This is a really unusual reaction."

I went to our pediatrician at the time and I said, "You need to help me. You need to help me figure out what's going on with my child." She referred me to a developmental psychologist. And she was the one who said, "I think he has sensory processing disorder," after we talked and she did her evaluation and I told her a lot of my concerns with his sensory issues, as well, with his getting upset about loud noises and bright lights and motions, and how he wasn't playing at the level that he should be. He should have been playing with his peers, and he was just playing by himself at preschool.

She sent him over to an occupational therapist, who did a full workup on him, did an evaluation on him. Sure enough, he was a couple of standard deviations behind in quite a few areas, developmentally. It was like, "Aha. At least I kind of know what I'm dealing with at this point."

Dara: Then what were the red flags looking back now? It's good for parents who are reading this to see, because everybody has different red flags. For me, Dylan had the yeast rash around his penis that wouldn't go away. He had the spitting up. He had the red cheeks that they kept telling me to put Aquaphor on, but it was food allergies. The drooling. The late walking and talking.

Maria: Initially it was colic, which gets brushed aside by pediatricians as, "Oh, all babies go through this. It's nothing to worry about." Colic, projectile vomiting, and acid reflux. He would take an hour to eat once we started him on solid food. He would eat five bites of food. I kept a spreadsheet on this, because I'm the analyst. Then he would throw it all up after every single meal. He did this for three and a half years, or so. He would throw up his food. They were like, "He doesn't have acid reflux. He just has a weak gag reflex." Because he wasn't eating enough, he developed failure to thrive. He went from the fiftieth percentile in weight at birth down to the third percentile at eighteen months.

It was only then that another pediatrician finally said, "Oh, wait. He's lost weight. Now we should listen to you." He then prescribed a fast food diet of french fries, chicken nuggets, and PediaSure. My older son lived on PediaSure for a couple years there. Of course, he would throw it all up. It definitely helped with his weight gain, but I cringe now when I look at the ingredients on the label. There's no way I would ever give this to anybody ever. It's full of, I believe, high-fructose corn syrup, or at least corn syrup solids, and genetically-modified foods. They throw vitamins on the label and make you think that those are good things that are in there, but those are actually synthetic vitamins. They're not the right form. It's not organic. It is just a big mess.

Then, like I said, the sensory issues, where we would go to the grocery store and five-ten minutes into it he'd just have a screaming fit. Everybody's looking at me like I'm a bad mom, and why can't you stop your baby from crying? It wasn't that. It was just that the sensory issues really got to him. When we'd take him to the playground, even when he was a small baby at about six months, when I put him on the swing he would cry. I'm like, "He's supposed to be enjoying this." I felt horrible, because all the other babies are having a great time and here he is crying on the playground equipment. He didn't like slides. He didn't like swings. He didn't like merry-go-rounds. He would just sit there and play by himself in the sand. I felt that that was just terrible and sad, because I didn't want my child to grow up without friends.

Dara: At what point did he actually get the diagnosis of SPD?

Maria: Just so you know, technically sensory processing disorder is not a "diagnosis" according to the DSM, the Diagnostic and Statistical Manual, so it's not covered by insurance. It was when he was about three and a half years old that he had the evaluation by the occupational therapist who said he has sensory processing disorder.

Dara: Then what did you do when you found that news out? Was it upsetting to hear that he had something that really you don't hear a lot about unless, of course you're in the autism community.

Maria: For me, it was helpful, because at least I knew what it was that we were dealing with. We started occupational therapy for him, which really helped a lot. It wasn't the end of everything, but it was definitely a good start.

Dara: What did you do next, besides the occupational therapy, and all the therapeutic interventions? How did you realize there was something wrong with his body?

Maria: It was really when I started working on my own health. I always tell people I got into this recovery issue backwards, because I didn't know at the time that sensory processing disorder was so much related to autism. I didn't know that kids could be recovered from it when he got his "diagnosis" of sensory processing disorder. Around the same time, I had started seeing a naturopath because of all the sensory issues that my son was dealing with. He would have temper tantrums and he was like a barnacle, he would just cry for hours and he was inconsolable. There was really nothing I could do to help him feel better, and it made me feel horrible as a mom to not be able to be there for my son. Then I had another son, as well, that I'm trying to deal with and he's got some issues of his own. It was extremely stressful.

All of a sudden, I developed middle-of-the-night insomnia, where I would wake up around one in the morning and not be able to go back to sleep for two or three hours. I would be dragging throughout the day, because I'm exhausted. I would take a nap but still be exhausted. I had severe adrenal fatigue. I developed shingles twice. I developed bronchitis, which I had never had before. I developed uterine fibroids, ovarian cysts, and an irregular cycle, which I had never had before. All of these things came within a six-month period.

I had gone to my regular gynecologist and he had given me Zoloft™ for the irritability and Ambien™ for an inability to sleep. The Ambien™ didn't help. The Zoloft™ helped take the edge off of things. I didn't like being on an antidepressant, so eventually I got off of it. I was very mainstream back then. I was like, "Well, this is what the doctor says, so let me try it." The Ambien™ didn't help. I was still waking up in the middle of the night for hours at a time. I'm like, "This is ridiculous." I finally started to say, "Well, maybe there's another answer out there." I started to do my own research, because that's what I do. I'm a research analyst.

I found out that magnesium could help. I'm like, "Well, hey. You know, it's a mineral. Why not? Give it a shot." I took the magnesium. Lo and behold, I started sleeping through the night. I went back to my gynecologist and I told him. He just shrugged his shoulders and said, "Whatever works for you." I'm like, "Holy cow. What else is out there that he's not telling me about if he just sort of blows this off?" I'm like, "This is earth-shattering. There are so many people that could be getting a great night's sleep if they just took magnesium."

Then I started to do my own research. I started to see a naturopath for myself for all the other issues that I had dealt with. He found out that I had heavy metal toxicity that was off the charts, as far as mercury and lead. I turned around and had my sons tested with a heavy metal hair test. My older son was at the 97th percentile for heavy metal toxicity. My younger son was at the 90th. I'm like, "Whoa. What else is going on with them?" I started to bring them in to see the naturopath, as well.

I guess one of the other red flags that I had forgotten to mention was that my older son also had asthma. It was so severe that he was on nebulizers. He was on Xopenex™. He was on steroids. He was on an inhaler. We had been in Los Angeles visiting my husband's family that summer. There were really bad forest fires in the San Gabriel Mountains. There was smoke pretty much the whole time we were there, that if you went outside you were breathing in. By the time we came back, after being there for a week, my son's asthma got really, really bad and he almost had to go to the hospital.

I brought him in to see our naturopath and he said, "Take him off of dairy." I'm like, "What?" Nobody had ever mentioned this, because we had been to one of the top allergists at Mount Sinai in New York. We had been to a pediatric gastroenterologist. None of our pediatricians had ever mentioned that. I'm like, "That's weird. Okay. I'll just go ahead and try it," because I had seen some good results for myself working with the naturopath. I'm like, "Okay. Let's just try it."

I take all dairy out. Lo and behold, he stops throwing up after every meal and stops needing the Prevacid™ that he had been taking for a while. I'm like, "Whoa. What's going on?" The asthma got better. I'm like, "Okay. There's stuff going on here that doctors aren't telling me about, and I'm starting to get really pissed off." I started to do more research, and of course continuing to take myself and the kids to the naturopath. Our health definitely improved, that's when I started to realize that it's not just the sensory issues, because taking out dairy helped with sensory issues as well. Then eventually I took out gluten, just because those two act in concert to cause so many health problems in a child.

That's when I realized that there was more than just that, and started to piece everything together, that it's what's going on underneath. It's the toxicity, gut dysbiosis, and immune dysregulation. It goes back to what Dr. Kenneth Bock wrote about in his book. Then tying it all together and doing even more research on my own. That's the impetus for the book that I wrote, *Almost Autism*; I wanted parents to have a roadmap and to be able to understand that it's not just that your child has autism. It's that he also has chronic constipation, which my kids had as well. They were on MiraLAX™ every single day. It's the chronic constipation. It's the chronic diarrhea. It's the dark circles under the eyes. It's the red cheeks or ears after eating. It's the bloated tummy. It's the chronic sniffly nose. It's the chronic ear infections.

It's all those red flags on top of the developmental delays, on top of the sensory issues, on top of, if your child has autism, being nonverbal or limited speech or limited social engagement. It's all tied together. Western medicine tends to see it as all separate things, Western medicine practitioners don't really tie it all together.

Dara: What would you say has helped your son the most?

Maria: Diet. Changing the diet, absolutely. I was part of the "Mothers Determined Panel" at the Autism One Conference in 2015, and also in 2016. We were all moms that have recovered our children. We've written books about it. We were selling our books at the conference, as well. People would come up and ask us, "What is the one thing that made the biggest difference?" Across the board, we all said, "Changing the diet. You gotta change the diet." A lot of people will say, "Well, you know, I tried the diet and it didn't work." Then you talk to them and they didn't do it one-hundred percent. Just because you try a diet, you need to try it for a while. If it's still not really making any difference, then I would say that there are probably other dietary things that you would need to dive into, as well, to go a little bit further into it.

It was really changing the diet for all of us. We saw such significant changes in our children and in the health of our children that it gave us a lot of momentum to keep going forward. Everything you read in the newspaper says diet makes no difference as far as a person's health. Then you do it yourself and you realize that it does. Maybe your child is sleeping better. Maybe he's not being as anxious. Maybe he's not being hyperactive. Maybe his allergies are better. Those kinds of things, you're like, "There's something to this and we should continue to explore this."

Dara: I know what you're saying when you say, "diet." Tell the readers when you say "diet," what type of changes do you mean?

Maria: The first diet most people do is to put their child on a gluten-free, dairy-free diet. Dairy includes all forms of dairy: cows milk, as well as sheeps milk, goat milk, whatever. That includes ice cream, yogurt, milk, cheese, anything that has dairy in it, even Goldfish Crackers. You've got to look at the label, the ingredient label, and make sure that that does not contain any of that potentially allergenic food in there. Like I said, going on the gluten-free, dairy-free diet is the starting diet for a lot of parents.

They can notice that their child isn't constipated anymore. Maybe the diarrhea gets better, that the child is able to focus better, have more attention. Some of their other symptoms start to go away, like the chronic ear infections, that's definitely tied to eating dairy.

Dara: Tell me about how your younger son was affected? He wasn't as affected as your older one with the SPD and the asthma and everything. Was it in softer ways?

Maria: Softer ways. He also had acid reflux. He also had developmental delays. He didn't walk until he was sixteen months old, which is still within the norm, but it's definitely more towards the outlier side of things. He had a slight vestibular issue, as well. For both of them, they would be sitting down in a chair at the kitchen table and they would just fall out of their chairs. Probably most parents would just say, "Well, that's weird," and laugh it off, and whatever, but that's a sign that the vestibular system is not working well and that child's sense of balance isn't working well, and that can have a huge impact as far as the developmental milestones that they go through, such as crawling and walking and those kinds of things.

I would take him swimming to Mommy and Me classes, where I'm holding onto him the whole time because he's a baby. He was about eighteen months old. He'd say, "I'm falling! I'm falling!" I'm like, "I'm holding you. You haven't even gone anywhere." We're just standing still in the pool, and he thinks he's falling, that says to me his vestibular system is out of whack. He benefited from me picking up on that and saying that there may be something just slightly off with him. He went through some of the therapy and some of the exercises that we did at home for his older brother and he's fine now.

Dara: So looking back, if you were just to rattle off a bunch of things that you think contributed that you just didn't know about at the time, what would they be? For instance, with Dylan, I could probably name twenty-five things that contributed including doing IVF and not knowing what's in all that stuff and my gut flora. I was very sick with an autoimmune at the time.

Maria: A lot of it starts with the mother, like you said. I can trace autoimmune diseases in my family, especially on the maternal side. Maternal stress, like I said, working on Wall Street, that played a huge factor as well. Then, there is maternal toxicity. A lot of people, even pediatricians, don't know that mothers pass on the toxicity to their babies, that's what the Environmental Working Group had written a landmark report about in 2005. It's called "Body Burden: The Pollution in Newborns." They showed that it was in the cord blood of these newborns, that there were an average of 200 different toxins and I believe 287 different toxins or toxicants, if you want to call them that, in the cord blood of a newborn, meaning that they could have only come from the mother.

So cleaning out and detoxing for the mother are huge. Stress, like I said and then, birth trauma and/or cesarean section can be a huge factor. Vaccines. I can tell you countless people, countless moms, whose children have regressed into autism after vaccines. For a lot of us, too, it's not that immediate regression that you can see. Sometimes it's just the slow disintegration of what they should have been and what they are now, that they didn't quite reach the potential that they should have. That's kind of hard to really put your finger on, especially as a new parent.

There are genetically modified foods in our diet. There are pesticides all over your foods, if you're not eating organic food that plays a huge part. There are toxins in our water, like fluoride and chlorine. We have artificial colors, artificial flavors, and preservatives in our food that cause a lot of problems, attention problems especially with our children.

Dara: What do you think is really important for parents to know who are trying to prevent autism?

Maria: I would say for the mother to seriously think about her health before she even decides to get pregnant. We're told to avoid fatty fish, because there could be mercury in there. Nobody's talking about the mercury that could be in you from the silver amalgams that have been in your mouth. So get the mother cleaned up as much as possible, be in a non-stressful state as much as possible during pregnancy. Make sure you're working with a naturopath or a functional medicine doctor to make sure that your thyroid and your adrenals are working well, because nobody really talks about how that affects the health of our children. That's what I found out both from myself and from my children, is that all three of us had adrenal and thyroid issues. That plays a huge role.

You'll want to make sure that you've had yourself tested for heavy metals as well as other sorts of toxins that could be in you. You may want to go through a really in-depth detox program, including far-infrared saunas. That would really help to detox and one of the best books I've read about that is *Detoxify or Die* by Sherry Rogers, MD.

Dara: I have that book on my shelf. I get her newsletter every month, too.

Maria: Doctors should read her book, it's a quick, easy read. She talks about how pretty much any disease or any disorder is caused by toxicity and nutritional deficiencies. I would add stress in there, too, as well as the gut dysbiosis.

Dara: You are a health coach. I am wondering if through all this trying to get yourself and your children healthier is the reason you became so interested and went for your certification?

Maria: Yes.

Dara: Please tell us about this.

Maria: I was working on Wall Street before this. I was popping ibuprofen every day and drinking lots of coffee and eating crappy microwaved food, my little Lean Cuisine microwave food.

Dara: Oh, god.

Maria: I was so healthy, right? I had no interest in this. I was doing fine. I was out buying lots of shoes and purses and all sorts of fun stuff, traveling, and just living the high life. It really was a good life. It wasn't until I had my own health problems and my kids' health problems too, that I really started to dig into this and figure out what's going on and thinking that, "Holy cow. We're being lied to about so many things." Industry has taken over regulation of itself, which is not a good situation when you have the fox guarding the hen house in regards to the FDA and the EPA and the CDC. You can't expect that industry is going to do a good job of policing itself.

A lot of what is out there is dictated to us through corporations in the guise of governmental agencies when, in fact, they're all in bed with each other. You have to really understand that if you want good health you can't just listen to the newspaper or the TV or the magazines. You actually have to go out and do your own research, talk with other parents. You want to read books, because books are not as censored and they're not paid for by corporations with advertising dollars. You can get a lot more unfiltered, uncensored information from books.

Dara: As a health coach and having two children with health issues that you've helped get better, do you think that there are things people can do to try to prevent autism?

Maria: Absolutely.

Dara: Do you work with families trying to prevent autism who already have a child with autism?

Maria: I think most people aren't thinking that far forward. It's usually you only deal with the situation when it's gotten so bad that you have to deal with it. That's just the way human nature is and that's how I was, and that's how most of us are. I know that a lot of people out there would love for moms to be thinking of true prevention. In all honesty, that usually doesn't happen. In my case, I'm actually dealing with parents who have children on the spectrum.

Dara: We talk a lot about soft signs in this book. What do you suggest a parent does if they see some of the soft signs?

Maria: I am also the media director and a board member for Epidemic Answers. It is a 501(c)(3) nonprofit. We put out a lot of great information. We let parents know what those soft signs are, and I wrote about it in my book, as well. If you just go to our website, which is www.epidemicanswers.org and look on there and you can see this whole list of some of the soft signs that I talked about. You can see that this could be your child. Your child may have some kind of chronic health condition and you may not have really pieced it together, because it's sort of the new norm for kids these days to all have EpiPens or inhalers or taking Zyrtec™ for their chronic drippy nose or their seasonal allergies.

Everybody's just in this haze and not really paying attention that our kids aren't healthy, especially when you look back at the health of how you were when you were a kid. It wasn't like this when we were kids.

Dara: If people go to the website that you just mentioned will they be able to look up practitioners that might be able to help them in the area that they live?

Maria: Yes. Absolutely. That's part of what I do is put together the practitioner database.

Dara: As a health coach and a parent, I want to ask you if you think parents really understand that the choices they make are incredibly important, especially when the kids are young?

Maria: I think we don't understand. I know I didn't, like all these horrible foods I was feeding my kids. Food is probably the most basic thing, as far as choice, and that you can do so much about. There's also a lot that you can do, as far as calming down the stressful environment that your family lives in.

You look at schools these days, or at least my kids' school, and they've got Smart Boards and they've got WiFi everywhere. These kids are being bombarded with EMF at school and at home. They're not being able to get into that proper state of rest and digest. They're all in a state of fight or flight. A body that is in a constant state of fight or flight is not able to heal and repair. As a parent, you can do so much to create a calming environment, slow down the pace of life. Maybe you don't run your kids around to soccer practice when they're young so much. You can work on those things when they're older.

You create a calming environment for sleep. You make sure that they're going to bed early. I find most kids these days, most of my sons' friends, they go to bed, in my mind, way too late. I'm thinking, "No wonder they've got behavioral problems," for one. There's tons that you can do that's in your control as a parent. A lot of it actually goes back to being what Patty Lemer calls being a cranky grandmother. Making sure the kids are going to bed early. Making sure that they're getting good, solid meals, not processed food, that's cooked at home with love by somebody.

I hate to say it, but I think a lot of that actually stems from dual-income parents, because there are both parents that are working. You farm out the responsibility to someone else of taking care of your child, I will tell you that nobody can take as good of care of your kid as you can. You're the best person for the job.

Dara: Do you think chronic illnesses such as autism can be reversed?

Maria: Yes. Absolutely. I've seen it in my own scope. I call sensory processing disorder almost autism. I've recovered my sons from it. I help parents recover their kids from it. I've got testimonials on my website. We have stories, real-life stories, on Epidemic Answers' website of kids who have recovered not just from autism but from ADHD, sensory processing disorder, asthma, allergies, OCD, and autoimmune diseases.

Dara: What do you hope people will take away from your story here today, which is just a much more brief version of your book that has tons of information about treating your children and what people can do?

Maria: I hope they take away hope that recovery is possible and that they should listen to themselves as parents, listen to that intuition inside of them that told them time and time again that something's wrong with their child, or maybe they shouldn't do this, or they got upset when the doctor didn't believe them or didn't agree with them. It's okay to leave a doctor or a pediatrician and go find somebody else that will listen to you. It's so important as a parent to be able to have that support group of like-minded parents. I hope that parents who read this come away with, because you have to know, that there's so much more out there that you are not being told that you really need to do your research and to find out.

Dara: How are your kids today?

Maria: They're really great. My older one is going into middle school. We're now dealing with not so much the sensory issues but the residual issues. That's what you'll find as you go through recovery. You're not just going to see, bam, one day your child is recovered from everything. It is still work. You still have to work off all the residual issues that you're dealing with. They're doing great in school. My younger son is in the gifted program at school. They've got lots of friends and they're happy kids. They're intelligent. They ask lots of questions. They're very sweet. They're very open. They're very empathetic. A lot of other parents have commented to me, especially about my older son, how it's such a nice thing to see that in another boy, to have a boy stick up for another, to be able to listen to him and hear him and calm him down, which is what my son does. I think that's just such a great testament to who he is. I'm very proud to be their mother. They're doing great.

✳ ✳ ✳

The only way to hear a child's journey with chronic illness is through their mother's lips. Any functional medicine doctor will tell you that it's the parents that are the driving force in this holistic movement. It is our unwavering determination and mission to bring our child's health back into balance that ultimately leads some of them down the path of recovery. Many parents who have a child with autism will spend hours upon hours researching everything from fixing mitochondrial dysfunction to dealing with an MTHFR mutation. We have been known to drive hundreds of miles just to buy a food that we instinctively know will help our child. I know this all sounds a little dramatic, but I promise you that it's not. Over the past ten years I have met astoundingly dedicated practitioners and parents.

These three moms are just a few examples of how incredibly thoughtful and special the parents of children who are sick with chronic illness can be. They persevere against every odd and don't take no for an answer that their child won't get better or recover. These parents not only fight for their child's health, but many of us must battle our city or state for an appropriate school program or exemption from vaccines that may have already injured our child's health. You cannot even begin to imagine the laundry list that a parent of a special needs child has on them at all times.

This brings me to one of the most important messages that I can leave parents with in this chapter, which is to make sure you take care of yourself too! Many of our children are what we call the canaries in the coal mine. They will succumb to the toxic effects of the surrounding environment first. But as the saying goes, the apple does not fall far from the tree. If you discover that you have a child with autism or any other chronic illness, then please take a long look at your own health. Many times the mother has the same underlying issues as the child even if it gets expressed into a "different" type of illness. That's why it is so important to make these changes to diet and lifestyle as a family, even if the initial reason is for the sick child. The whole family will benefit from green cleaning products, less EMFs, and an organic whole foods diet. I found it to be very convenient to do to myself whatever I was trying with Dylan whether it was a special diet, probiotic, or even IV vitamin C. We both definitely benefited from everything we did.

And if you are someone who is reading this book who has not had a baby yet, then you are the luckiest person around. You can only imagine how much I wish that I knew this information that I have today before Dylan was born. If there was ever one wish I could be granted, it would be to go back in time and do it all over for him. Sadly you know I can't. But what I have done is create a beautiful and hopefully lasting legacy for him. This book is Dylan's legacy. I am just the medium for his message. It is through his painful journey that others will be able use this information that we have learned along the way to prevent autism and other childhood chronic illnesses in their own child.

I cannot express how thankful I am to Corinne, Katie, and Maria for their willingness to share their stories with all of you. The information that they have shared is both eye-opening and thought provoking. I only hope that you are half as inspired by them as I am. My goal was to honor each one of the children featured in this chapter by allowing their story to be told, so they could help other children, and their suffering would not be in vain.

A special thanks to Patrick, Christian, and Ryan; you are all such beautiful children and greatly loved by many.

Chapter 13

MY KITCHEN

I think it's really important for me to spend some time speaking about how you can get started on making better choices. One thing every practitioner in this book agrees on is that nutrition is paramount when it comes to prevention. I personally know just how downright daunting the task of making these changes will be for some people, which is why I devote this entire chapter to the subject. I will never forget feeling like a deer in the headlights when I came home from that very first appointment with Dr. Nancy O'Hara and had the tall task of implementing this gluten- and dairy-free diet that was completely foreign to me at the time. However, I quickly learned that better choices and healing almost always start in your kitchen. Remember how Maria mentioned that parents who were successful in getting their children better unanimously agreed that the single most important thing that helped their child was improving their diet. So if this is what can bring a person back from a state of disease, then wouldn't it make sense that it would have an easier time of preventing one in the first place? I thought the best way to help spur your imagination or get you over the hesitating hump would be to take you through my own kitchen evolution, this way you have an example on which to base how one makes these changes.

My kitchen today has no resemblance to the kitchen I had over ten years ago before Dylan was diagnosed. I assumed that if it was sold in a store that it was safe. And the word "natural" meant to me that all the ingredients were wholesome and from nature. I started to have a little bit of a wake-up call when I got pregnant with my son. My husband and I began to purchase some organic food as it was becoming a little more popular. Whole Foods may have even just opened in NYC. And then after my son was born, I tried to make sure everything we bought was organic for him, but not necessarily for my husband and I. Due to convenience and our lack of culinary skills, we were still ordering up food from restaurants four times a week and eating most daytime meals from a deli. Of course, I cringe when I think back to my eating habits, but they were far worse when I was a teenager and a single person in my twenties.

When I look back at my childhood, it's not that difficult to pinpoint where the first seed towards a healthy lifestyle was planted. My upbringing was a little unusual compared to a lot of my friends. I had friends whose mothers cooked everything from scratch, and then knew others who were given a lot of junk food. My mom wasn't even in between. She used to take us to a health store to do the majority of her shopping a few months out of the year, buying natural soda and freshly ground peanut butter. Then there were those months that she would bring us to a regular supermarket, allowing my brother and me to put anything our hearts desired in the shopping cart, including Captain Crunch cereal, Snickers bars, and Fudgsicles. I never questioned her extreme flip-flop, since it was this way for as long as I could remember. As an adult, I now look back and think it had something to do with her mental state and/or the fact that she might have been trying the latest fad diet. My mother suffered from both major depression and borderline personality, which means she had both the psychological and physical effects of mental illness. She also had gut dysbiosis as well as food allergies, which would make her break out in hives on her face whenever she ate strawberries or tuna fish. You cannot even imagine how much I wish she was still around, so I could bring her to a functional medicine doctor to fix the part of the depression that was caused by toxins and her gut issues.

I feel fortunate that I was exposed to buying food from a health store decades before it became popular, and equally happy that I never took on her extreme behavior towards food. I believe this early influence ignited some kind of passion inside of me long before my son's autism. I remember that I used to sit in the waiting room at a doctor's office as a teenager and read any health magazine that was available. I just had an innate interest. But I still did not understand the concept of how important diet was in preventing illness and how the food you ate could cause illnesses over time. This view might be a result of the fact that my parents had a phone book just for doctors. It actually said "Doctors" on the cover. They were very adamant about going to the "best" doctors for every problem that they had. A new pill or procedure was revered as the greatest thing. Luckily I also came from a family lineage that is very sensitive to pharmaceuticals in the way of adverse reactions, so I did not take a lot of them.

I ate a lot of fast food, since my mom would go through these "dark spells" where she was moody and did not want to cook. Looking back she probably just couldn't bring herself to. My brother and I had our share of Carvel, pizza,

Kentucky Fried Chicken, Arthur Treacher's, you name it, we probably ate it. But somehow I don't think the food was nearly as toxic as it is today. They just didn't have the same chemicals and preservatives available that we do now. As Geri Brewster mentioned in her chapter, a piece of pizza just isn't a piece of pizza anymore. Many times it's a toxic soup of chemicals, which will have some unknown effect on our body.

Luckily for Dylan, my husband and I did not eat fast food that often or drink soda by the time he was born and he never consumed either of those things. However, we would make him chicken nuggets that came from a store-bought box, or cook mac and cheese made from both organic milk and cheese slices. So I guess things could have been worse, but I certainly wish I knew more at the time. Dylan displayed food allergy symptoms right from the get go, and unsurprisingly his regular pediatrician never figured it out. Unfortunately, there is so much that mainstream doctors just still do not get. They are literally taught to give a prescription for almost any symptom you have, rather than look for the actual cause. Hence the reason I call it band-aid medicine.

It is sad to me that most people don't understand that if you keep taking a pill to mask a symptom then the situation will most likely just get worse over time, since you are not dealing with the imbalance or deficiency in the body which is causing the symptom in the first place. Now I do want to point out that I am not against western medicine. There is certainly a time and a place for it. If I was ever in a serious car accident, there is nowhere else I would want to be than in a Level 1 trauma center. An equally important situation would be if someone is in heart failure and needs immediate surgical intervention. All the green juice and gluten-free bread in the world isn't going to get them out of that emergency situation.

But then you have the droves of people who take pharmaceutical interventions for just about everything under the sun. Unfortunately, I believe that my mom had this blind trust in medicine that ultimately led to her untimely death. I will tell you her story just so you can see how when things go wrong they can go really wrong.

It all started when my mom had a hysterectomy for some fibroids about a year before her death, since that was the gold standard of care back in the eighties. They still do it today, but also have other options as well. As some of you may know, you go into menopause immediately following a hysterectomy, and these sudden hormone changes seemed to exacerbate her already existing mental illness. I imagine that she was also psychologically coping with the fact that her womanhood was taken from her. In any event, she became much more depressed afterwards and had the wherewithal to check herself into an inpatient institution in Hartford, Connecticut. She was also seeing a psychiatrist in New York City. Her doctors put her on all kinds of new antidepressants including an SSRI that I believe might have been in the experimental stage at the time when she took it. My mom left the institution after being very unhappy with the level of care she was receiving and came home in early August that year. She was still taking medication and I watched in horror as she tried to kill herself every day for twenty-three days straight until she finally succeeded in hanging herself. Mind you she had never attempted suicide before this time and had battled depression all her life. In those three weeks, I saw things no child should ever have to witness. Not only did I come home to find her, untie the noose, and take her down, but I had already witnessed twenty-three days straight of all the different ways one can try to kill themselves. I will never know whether the final act or the twenty-three days caused me to eventually be diagnosed with PTSD. I am happy to report that I no longer suffer from the PTSD that caused those terrible nightmares for the next seventeen years following her death.

I truly believe that she did not have to die. Nobody will ever convince me that she got the best possible care that she deserved. Her psychiatrist was away for the month of August, so she probably had nobody to tell that she was having increased suicidal thoughts and ideation. Today there is a black box warning that is now placed on any SSRI prescription bottle citing the possibility of these symptoms occurring. This experience with my mom's death swayed me from mainstream medicine and certainly any pharmaceuticals that have a direct effect on the brain. Please don't misconstrue that I think all pharmaceuticals are bad. Overall they just are not good for people who have very sensitive chemistry like my family. I realize many pharmaceuticals keep people alive who may otherwise have died, including antidepressants. However, I also know with one-hundred-percent certainty that my mom would have fared much better being treated with a functional medicine doctor who understood her underlying condition and the symptoms that it was causing.

My diet continued on a downward spiral after she died. It really hit rock bottom once we got a microwave the following year and started melting fake chemical food into plastic containers that came with them. My father did not cook at all and found it easiest to purchase and give us food that came from a box, which was becoming much more readily available. It was around this time I remember starting to not feel that great. I noticed my belly was bloated and I was constipated a lot of the time. So I ignored it like most teenagers would. It wasn't until the anxiety developed that I started to try to take better care of myself and began buying my food in the same health food store that my mom took me to when I was a little girl. I still continued to eat out with friends and purchase my share of junk food. There just wasn't a full connection yet to the idea that food is so important and how dangerous the chemicals and preservatives in some processed food can be. It would be another couple decades before I grasped this important basic understanding of "real or true" health.

So now that you have a little bit of my history, it's easy to understand how I jumped head-first into trying to heal my son with diet and natural interventions. I never imagined how much changing our diet would help my own health. I didn't realize it at the time but I had terrible allergies when I was trying to get pregnant with my son. As I've said, I believe my body was not healthy enough to get pregnant, which is why we needed to do IVF. But it was Dylan's diagnosis that ultimately led us down the path to where we are today. Right after the diagnosis, I went home and researched everything I could to find out about autism, even though that neurologist gave me the bleak "there is nothing you can do" speech. I immediately read all about the GFCF diet helping lots of kids. So when we had our appointment with Dr. Nancy O'Hara I was armed and ready when she told me to implement that diet immediately. I started the very next day. I won't pretend that it was not difficult. It's kind of like trying to take a crash course in learning a new language. But I remember thinking, nothing I could do, no matter how inconvenient, would ever compare to how gut wrenching it is to watch your child slip away into the depths of autism.

At first the diet seemed easy enough, since I just had to buy food that had gluten and dairy-free written on the label. However as I got more engulfed in the diet, I noticed it wasn't that simple after all. I began to learn that gluten could be hidden in almost anything, including salt. Many times the word "natural flavors" or "natural spices" can actually mean that gluten is in the product. So you cannot just go by reading ingredients alone. And if you are super sensitive like me and the product is made in a facility that also produces other products with wheat, then you may have a problem with the cross contamination that can occur. You really have to become a private detective to do the diet correctly. People just don't understand that you cannot put gluten-free bread in a toaster that had regular bread in it, since the cross contamination is enough to give the body a reaction. This is why I believe many people try the diet and say it didn't help at all. Some people do give it an honest effort, but don't comprehend how you cannot even have a bite of a cookie that has gluten in it. The bite of the cookie will stay in your blood for thirty days. The other thing is that sometimes it can take being on the diet for months to feel a positive difference.

People seem to expect some miraculous reaction. I once spoke to someone who did the gluten-free diet for months and said she felt better but nothing crazy. I asked her what she noticed. Funny enough, she rattled off a pretty long list of improved memory, no more mental fog, a lot less constipated, better energy and so on. I immediately started laughing and asked her what were you expecting, you named some nice improvements that anyone would like to have. I think she had an "Aha" moment right there in front of me and said, "You're right, I did feel a ton better. I am going back on the diet tomorrow!"

Now not everyone has to go gluten-free to be healthy, although it is considered a very inflammatory food. One of the most famous experts in the world on gluten, as Dr. Baker points out, is Alessio Fasano, who states that only one food opens the tight junctions in everyone's intestines: gluten. He further explains why some people don't have a problem with it and others will has to do with how long the junctions stay open. This is based on an individual's body chemistry. But the fact remains that it is a very inflammatory food that seems to be harder for people to digest, which may be caused by how it's grown, treated, and processed these days.

I will never forget my own experience of how I first learned how much I was affected by gluten. Shortly after my husband and I put Dylan on a gluten- and dairy-free diet, we joined him and went on it too. It just seemed to make the most sense so that the kitchen would not have cross contamination. I was on the diet for three months, at which time we went away on vacation to Montauk. I made a conscious decision that I would cheat a little when we went out to eat at some of my favorite restaurants. And one day I was sitting on the beach reading Star Magazine and I noticed that I had to read the same sentence over and over again about some celebrity getting busted for drugs. I took note and said to myself, "What is wrong with me?" since for the past few months my brain had been so clear. I immediately made the connection that for the past week I was eating gluten, so I stopped right at that very moment. It took a few weeks of not eating gluten but my mental clarity returned and I never purposely ingested it again. And I noticed a ton of other symptoms that improved over the years such as my memory, word recall, and energy level. I started to be able to read books for the first time in my life, since I experienced such horrible reading comprehension difficulties. It is now apparent to me that I suffered from a gluten disability during all my formative school years. Somehow my short-term memory was not affected, so I was able to memorize things well enough to pass quizzes and tests. Again, I don't think everyone has to go gluten free, but if you have a child that is really struggling in school then I would certainly give it a try. And most people think that you have to rely on blood test results on whether or not to take it out. Dr. Nancy O'Hara was the first person to tell me that there is no better test than just taking it out for a period of time and I could not agree more with this statement.

I personally have intentionally avoided eating gluten for the past ten years. However, there have been times when I have gone out to eat and no matter how careful I am, I know that I was accidentally given gluten. I try to go to restaurants with gluten-free menus since they seem to be more careful and aware of food allergies. Sometimes you just get stuck with a meal that has gluten in it from cross contamination in the kitchen. The symptoms usually appear within an hour or two and continue for two to five days. I am affected by gluten neurologically, although I do get really constipated by it as well. You can give me a magazine to read and I can literally tell you an hour and a half after a meal if it had gluten in it. Unfortunately, the distinction is that dramatic. And I want to add that I always take digestive enzymes when I am eating out at a restaurant. I do this not just for the gluten, but for all the other stuff, which might be in the food they prepare that my body is not used to.

At home my husband and I cook with the cleanest and purest ingredients. The type of cooking that we do now definitely evolved from one type of diet in particular: the Specific Carbohydrate Diet (SCD). We decided to embark on the SCD diet after Dylan was doing the GFCF diet for about nine or ten months and we weren't really seeing any of the dramatic or positive effects that we had hoped for. I began to research what other diets and biomedical treatments were out there for us to try. Somehow I kept coming across the SCD diet, which was being touted as a gut healing diet. By this time, I vaguely understood how much disease and more notably autism occurs when the gut is not healthy.

Our functional medicine doctor, Nancy O'Hara, was a little surprised when I told her that I was going to try the SCD diet on Dylan, since it wasn't nearly as popular as the GFCF at the time. Little did I know how much harder this diet would prove to be. You literally have to cook every single meal and morsel of food that you eat from scratch. Not only that, but every ingredient you use has to be a monosaccharide. This meant that you were giving up all grains and complex carbohydrates, which even included root vegetables. There would also be no dairy or sweetener other than honey used. It is basically the caveman diet consisting of meat, fruit, vegetables and nuts. There is an introductory phase where you eat a lot of cooked fruits and drink bone broth. However, we just dove in and did the best that we could. I was very excited to try this diet, hoping it would get rid of some yeast that I knew I had. This diet proved to be miraculous for me. After six weeks, I noticed that my allergies were down by seventy percent, which is why I stayed on it for three more years. Dylan did not show the kind of improvements that I did, but he was markedly calmer on the diet, and I knew that he wasn't continuing to be harmed by the chemicals and preservatives in his food.

As you learned, nutrition is one area that all the practitioners interviewed for this book agree is vital in preventing chronic illness and helping a child improve from one as well. For that reason I am going to go through some of the specific categories that they believe each of us need to pay close attention to in order to greatly reduce our child's risk of autism.

ORGANIC

We know that just living near an area that is sprayed with pesticides can increase the chance your child will be diagnosed with autism. So wouldn't it make sense that not eating pesticides would be a good idea too? However it doesn't just stop there. The lack of pesticides and chemicals sprayed on food while it's grown is just one benefit that organic food has over conventional food. When pesticides aren't used the soil is healthier, since the good microbes that inhabit the field have not been killed. Many times the food that is yielded by organic farming has higher levels of nutrients when it is not grown in mineral depleted soil. Many people cannot afford organic food as it can be more expensive. There are ways to work around this problem such as purchasing food in bulk, buying from a CSA, or buying frozen fruits and vegetables. Then there is a list of the "clean fifteen" that the Environmental Working Group produces every year that shows the nonorganic fruits and vegetables that are sprayed less and safer to eat if you are buying conventionally raised produce. You can find this list as well as the dirty dozen fruits and vegetables that are the most heavily sprayed conventional fruits and vegetables that is consistently updated on the Environmental Working Group's website: www.ewg.org

HEALTHY FATS

Sadly people have become quite phobic to eating fats. Meanwhile they could not be a more important part of a healthy diet especially for a growing child. Your brain needs fat to function well. Picking your fats is equally important to eating them. You need to be careful of which ones you choose to cook with though as they can structurally change due to high heat and become carcinogenic. Fats that are safe for high heat cooking are coconut oil, duck fat, palm oil, ghee, and avocado oil. I use the omega 6 vegetable oils sparingly as they are very inflammatory. However I would use organic canola oil to fry something from time to time. In general I put olive oil on all my food that is not cooked on a high heat. Some people also do very well using nut oils.

One big reason it is so important to eat healthy fat with each meal is that it's what keeps you from being hungry. When you consume a carbohydrate with fat, it does not allow your blood sugar to spike. There has been a lot misinformation that consuming fat will make you gain weight. It is sugar and complex carbohydrates that are the problem. I make sure my children eat plenty of fat and protein all the time.

GRAINS AND "NON GRAINS"

You have heard countless times throughout the book that gluten is very inflammatory. However too many grains, regardless of whether they are gluten-free or not, can be equally damaging to your gut. Your bad bacteria likes to feast on excess sugar that can come from too many carbs that ferment in your gut. It is a great idea to stick with the gluten-free grains as often as possible, and they could not be easier to find. People are also catching on to the fact that many of the "non-grain grains" are not only gluten-free but quite healthy. Many of them contain a lot of minerals and protein. Some that I particularly like are: quinoa, millet, buckwheat, and teff. They all cook very similarly to rice.

When I do prepare regular grains, I make sure they are the whole grain, which means it is eaten from its original state and minimally processed, such as sweet potatoes. I will also soak my rice or purchase it sprouted. This way it has been predigested, which is healthier for your gut. It is very easy to soak your grains, all you have to do is place them in water with a little bit of acid such as lemon or ½ teaspoon of raw apple cider vinegar. You leave it out on the counter for eight hours, rinse it thoroughly and then cook as desired. This can be done easily with rice or quinoa. Root vegetables are also nice to use in place of complex carbohydrates since they are packed with wonderful phytonutrients.

FERMENTED FOODS

Please do not underestimate how important feeding your microbiome the right kind of food is to keeping healthy bacteria in check. Fermented foods are very important to implement in your child's diet alongside a good probiotic. You can do this with fermented vegetables or with a nicetasting fermented beverage. Letting your child decide helps them feel that they are taking an important part in their health. These days it is very easy to purchase well-made fermented foods. Don't confuse regular pickles that contain vinegar with ones naturally fermented using sea salt such as Bubbies, which are sold almost everywhere. Other brands I like are Real Pickles and Hawthorn Valley, both of which can be purchased from a Whole Foods and most health food stores. It is also quite easy to make them yourself. A lot of kids enjoy fermented carrots and ginger or beets. Fermented drinks like Beet Kvass or Coconut Kefir are also quite palatable for children. My daughter even enjoys drinking the brine from the pickle jar since it is pretty salty. My advice would be to start them out early so it becomes an integral part of their diet.

GENETICALLY MODIFIED FOOD

This is a really important area to pay attention to. GMOs have been introduced into our food supply with no long-term studies. Scientists have no idea what the implications will be on our long-term health in the future. They can be dangerous to people who have food allergies as they can splice a gene from seafood for instance and put it in a tomato. Then some unsuspecting person eats the tomato and can have a severe reaction. This is just one of the potential dangers, and there are many others including studies on rats that showed they produced multiple tumors in just a few months of eating genetically modified food. You have also heard from many of the practitioners that the GMO food allows them to spray enormous amounts of pesticides such as Roundup without killing the crop, which means you are feeding your family even more chemicals. Ideally it is best to buy organic, however that may be out of the economic reach for some people. Again, you may have to be a little bit creative in order to eat healthy. Sometimes joining a CSA or volunteering your time for one will make it more economical, or purchasing frozen organic vegetables. You can try growing your own food if you have the land to do it. This would be my favorite option, as I would know every little thing about the way it was produced and handled.

At the very least try to stay away from buying non-organic of the most heavily produced GMO food: corn, soy, cottonseed, and canola. Remember that most processed food contains GMO unless it says non-GMO or organic. For example they use GMO sugar beets to produce sugar for many processed food products as well as genetically modified high fructose corn syrup. Even if it's not organic, the product needs to say cane sugar for you to know that it's not made with GMO sugar beets. I would do your absolute best to stay away from anything genetically modified, otherwise you will just be playing a part in this vast human experiment that is going on.

PROCESSED FOOD

I prefer to stay away from food that comes in a bag or a box with lots of ingredients on the list as much as possible. There are plenty of times that I buy my share of popcorn, potato chips, and cookies for my kids to enjoy. However I am just really careful about which companies' products I buy. It is a lot easier these days to find good quality processed food than it was years ago. Try to imagine that if you don't understand or cannot pronounce a chemical or preservative, then there is a good chance your body won't know what to do with it either. It can inhibit proper digestion, stay in your body and add to your toxic load.

GLASS KITCHENWARE

Many of the practitioners have mentioned that they think a big cause for fertility problems and early puberty has to do with all the endocrine disruptors that come from plastic products that we use everyday. We think nothing of drinking water from plastic bottles all day long, heating food up and storing it in plastic. There are a lot of things you can do to minimize these hormone disruptors. It is so easy to buy glass storage jars. They are not that expensive and tend to last much longer than the plastic ones without yellowing. My entire family uses glass water bottles with a silicone sleeve so it has less of a chance of breaking if it's accidentally dropped. They even make ones with a straw for the kids. And we purchase five-gallon jugs of water that come to our house in glass from Mountain Valley Spring Water. Another great choice is to buy a good quality water filter and you can save money over time on the endocrine disrupting plastic water bottles besides protecting your health.

PLASTIC WRAP AND TINFOIL

I find both of these to be dangerous when they touch your food day after day. I have Ziploc bags in my house, but my food does not touch the plastic. We use brown parchment paper, which even comes in a sandwich bag size to wrap up most of our food. Then I may put it in a Ziploc bag if the item needs to be airtight. I never use tinfoil anymore except once a year at Thanksgiving and I cover the turkey first in parchment paper so the tinfoil does not have the ability to touch and leech into my food. Recently a cousin of mine showed me her bloodwork that had extremely high levels of mercury and aluminum. She asked for my help in trying to figure out how she was coming in contact with so much heavy metals. I asked her a bunch of questions that allowed me to determine that the mercury was most likely from eating fish five nights a week and the aluminum probably came from the fact that she was heating up three meals a day every day using aluminum foil.

BABY FORMULA AND FOOD

Many of the baby formula manufacturers now produce an organic version of their formulas, however when I looked at the label I still could not understand more than half the ingredients on the list. For this reason, I would never have the confidence to feed that to my baby. As I mentioned, I breastfed for as long as I could and supplemented with the homemade Weston Price Foundation recipe that was extremely nutrient dense. I understood every ingredient that I was placing in that formula and there were absolutely no preservatives or chemicals. The recipe for the homemade formula was a little daunting to put together at first, but I quickly got used to making it. My husband and I used to make ten quarts at a time, and the freezer became our good friend. We made a large batch and froze enough so we would not have to make it too often. It may not be as convenient as buying a bottle of ready-made formula but I knew that I was giving my daughter something very nourishing.

The supplements that we decided to give right when she came home from the hospital were infant probiotic if she was not breastfeeding and getting it from me, vitamin D, 5-MTHF (the right kind of folate), B12, fish oil, and cod liver oil. All of these were ultimately placed in the homemade baby formula that she took in order to supplement breastfeeding.

We also prepared all her baby food from scratch, which is especially easy now that they sell all the gizmos you could possibly need to do it seamlessly, including a baby food blender and silicone freezer trays to save what you make in small amounts. This way you take one cube out of the silicone tray at a time. You just have to think ahead and get in the habit of putting it in the fridge the night before or leaving it out in the morning. Occasionally I bought the organic baby food puree in glass jars from the store when I ran out. But most important I was very careful not to introduce grains until she was at least a year old and I started with the "non-grain" grains. I am proud to say that my daughter has never been given gluten, soda or any fast food. This is not to say that I don't allow her to have the healthy version of junk food, especially in social situations, such as popcorn, potato chips, gluten-free pretzels, sorbet, and chocolate. I am just very careful about balancing the amount of carbs and sugar that she consumes. So for instance if she had eaten a lot of junk on a particular day at a birthday party or holiday then I would try to make up for it by being especially vigilant the next day. So I don't want to come off like some perfect mom, since

I do let her live a little. We just try to be very careful with her given the genetics that are already stacked against her.

BONE BROTH

We know that the health of a person's microbiome is the biggest predictor of whether or not they will suffer from a serious illness. It takes effort to keep it healthy, especially given how toxic our environment is today. I am of the belief that we need to constantly be detoxing and healing our digestive tracts just to stay one step ahead of disease. My husband I put forth a lot of effort in trying to feed our kids foods that will nourish their microbiome. Bone broth is extremely healing for the digestive tract and we serve it most mornings in our home. You can drink a cup any time of day as a snack, prior to or with a meal. Once you are able to get over your preconceived idea of what a meal should look like you will be a lot better off. I will always remember Dr. Nancy O'Hara telling me that you need to eat your dinner for breakfast. What she meant is that the body needs protein, not a muffin when you wake up. And she is exactly right. Bone broth is a soothing way for your digestive tract to start it's day. It is quite simple to make from scratch and the extra portions can easily be frozen. However there are many food companies that produce healthy versions that can be purchased in a health food store or certain supermarkets.

FRESH HERBS

Another culinary method I use to promote a healthy gut is to put fresh herbs on our food. My son loves fresh rosemary and oregano especially on a big, fat grass-fed steak. Herbs are wonderful for your health and so easy to keep around. I have to be a little bit more sneaky with my daughter, since she does not like seeing big pieces of green herb on her food. Many herbs also have multiple uses, for example rosemary and oregano have antimicrobial properties, so they can help kill the bad germs in your belly. Some of these are anti-inflammatory and the list of benefits goes on. I use herbs in tinctures as an antibiotic treatment, which you will learn about in the next chapter, My Natural Medicine Cabinet. You should try to use herbs on your food as often as possible. Not only are they health promoting but they make your food taste great too.

GETTING YOUR CHILD TO EAT NEW FOODS

My son and daughter have a very different approach to food. Sometimes I get lucky that Jessica just likes something healthy; other times she has to be either bribed or talked into how good it is for her. You need to find the tactic that works for your individual child. Dylan could never be bribed into taking something that he didn't want to. But lucky for me he allows me to give him some of the most awful tasting herbs and food he does not want under the premise that it will help him get better. When I explain that concept, he will inevitably take anything I give him, since he desperately wants to get better, especially back when he still could not speak.

With Jessica it is different, since she is more of a typical child. I used to bribe her at first to try something, then it moved into, "You have to take four bites or you don't get dessert." Now it's easier that it has been going on for so long, since we talk about natural medicine in my home on a near constant basis. One thing that got her very interested in vegetables is when she was three years old, I used to let her make her own salad with a butter knife.

Be creative and take advantage of any opportunity that encourages them to eat healthier. My kids come home from school each day and have a salad as a snack while they wait for me to cook dinner. I know this sounds funny that a salad isn't really considered a snack. Well for most people chicken soup isn't breakfast either. As I mentioned, you will probably need to abandon some of your old ways of thinking as you take on a healthier lifestyle. I definitely did and now don't give it a second thought to carry around a big container of bacon if we have to go to a doctors appointment for instance. And I always have jars of cut up fruits and vegetables if we are out at the park or playground. A big treat for my daughter on any given day is a B12 lollipop. Children are adaptable but they need for you to be confident in your food choices, then it will be easy for them to follow suit.

The most important advice that I can give is to tell you not to beat yourself up for what you have not done yet. Tomorrow is always a new day. And even though today you may have had a bad meal, you can always strive to make the next one better. The reason I included this chapter about my evolution is that I was hoping it may inspire you, so you don't get intimidated and try to do everything perfectly at once. You can't expect to build this new healthy lifestyle overnight. My hope is also that you will not give up even if it doesn't come so easy to you at first. Just try to make a few small changes and over time you will gradually see your own household evolve into something completely different.

Now that I have touched on some of my favorite health promoting foods that are so good for you, I would like to mention some that I don't care for. There are ingredients in some so called health foods that I stay clear away from. One of the reasons I don't buy the alternative milks such as hemp, almond, or coconut milk from the store is that many of them contain guar gum or xantham gum. I find these ingredients can be detrimental to a gut you are trying to heal. They can cause problems for many people. I would rather make these milks myself or pay extra to have it made fresh somewhere else. Some cold cuts also contain another ingredient I am not fond of called carrageenan. And there are cold cut companies that don't use the carrageenan, such as Nuna Naturals. One other notable mention is that there is confusion that natural nitrates like celery root are completely safe, and this isn't true. Many times they use a lot more of the celery root powder since it is considered "natural" and it can be even worse for you. So you really need to educate yourself on the food you buy. It's definitely worth doing a little bit of investigating. I find it easiest to sign up for some newsletters from reputable people and companies that do the research for me in a nice tightly written article. I will list some of my favorites in the back of the book such as ones from Russell Blaylock, MD, and Sherry Rogers, MD.

One of the best things that you can do to get started on a healthier way of life is to lower the amount of processed food you eat. This way you will automatically get rid of the chemicals and preservatives that will disrupt your digestive system and add to your total load. Staying away from genetically modified food should also be a priority. I don't know about you, but I am not interested in being part of this human experiment. I look for food that is organic or at least says non-GMO. Just remember that the idea of buying organic and not eating processed food is that you want to stop adding to the body's toxic load. All of this will take a little bit of trial and error to figure out the things that will work for you. I am constantly striving to make improvements and additions to my own kitchen preparations and traditions. It's an ongoing evolution, luckily one that I truly enjoy.

There is quite a large crossover between food and natural medicine when you really get into it. I find one ultimately always leads into the other. There are many foods and herbs that you both eat and use to treat certain conditions. This is an area that I have become extremely passionate about and fond of; the entire next chapter is devoted to this very concept. I hope you have found this condensed version of my own history and evolution to be helpful in finding and creating your own.

CHAPTER 14

MY NATURAL MEDICINE CABINET

I t has taken me years to get to the point where I do not feel the need to call a doctor to treat most everyday illnesses. The best explanation that I can give you is that I have been playing the role of doctor for ten years now. Many parents who have a child with autism will tell you that they feel this way too. For me I just got tired of going to the doctor for minor ailments and always being met with a prescription for some drug or product that potentially had some very serious or significant side effects. As I mentioned earlier that my family has a long list of people who have experienced adverse reactions to pharmaceutical products, so my feeling has always been why take the chance for such a minor ailment. So I was given no choice but to explore alternative natural treatments for each of these issues as they arose. Our functional medicine practitioners have been extremely helpful in this process.

Dr. Nancy O'Hara was one of my family's first biomedical doctors to prescribe natural herbal supplements to treat a wide variety of issues that Dylan had experienced. I will never forget the "Aha" moment I had when she suggested garlic and mullein drops to treat a minor ear infection. A light bulb literally went off inside my head or at least that is what I visualize happened, when I discovered that pharmaceutical drugs and over the counter medicines were not the only choice.

I consider my journey down this path of natural medicine to be one of the most rewarding things I have ever done with my time. People who know me really well can tell you that I am extremely passionate about holistic medicine— and that would probably be putting it lightly. I am very excited at the prospect of sharing some tips that I have discovered along the way for treating common everyday illnesses to get you on the road to building your own natural medicine cabinet. And who knows, maybe this chapter will spark a flame in one of you to continue traveling down this path too.

In the beginning of our journey, I just followed our biomedical doctor's instructions on what to do to try to improve Dylan's health. I was of course entering this new world that I refer to as functional or holistic medicine. I use these terms interchangeably. Years later, this morphed into a collaboration between our practitioners and I deciding together, since I recognized early on that he did not respond well to pharmaceutical drugs. For this reason, I centered my focus on researching and studying natural supplements that could help heal his body. I can confidently say that I now have pretty extensive knowledge of natural supplements. One of my favorite pastimes is to read articles and books on natural herbs to understand how they might help heal specific organs and the body as a whole. I now tend to call up our functional medicine practitioners with a list of supplements that I would like to try and explain why I want to use them. This way I get to bounce the idea off someone extremely intelligent to make sure it is both safe and appropriate, as well as obtain the correct dosage. It is through working on one of the most complex illnesses that I gained a lot of confidence to treat the minor ailments that one seems to come across, most often with their children.

As you read in my disclaimer, nothing you read in this chapter should be construed as medical advice. You will need to consult with your own child's practitioner before trying any of these natural remedies to see if they are appropriate specifically for your child. Dr. O'Hara was one of the first people to plant the seed of holistic medicine that eventually has become such a big part of my life. I feel very thankful that we were led to her so early on after Dylan's diagnosis. She helped us learn how to use many different natural medicines, and it has proven to be extremely helpful to Dylan and my family over the years.

So let's start with some of my most favorite items that can sit in your natural medicine cabinet for a very long time and be used to treat a variety of different complaints. I like to say that if I was ever stranded on a deserted island and could only have a few things at my finger tips, they would most certainly be raw apple cider vinegar, sea salt, and manuka honey. These three items can be used to treat a wide array of minor ailments. Let's go through some of the most common conditions that both children and adults seem to get, and I will explain how I have successfully treated them with natural substances.

Ear Infections: These can be quite painful and many times can be caused by a virus. For this, I will give my children one teaspoon twice a day of liquid elderberry to treat the part that may be caused by a virus. Elderberry is one of the strongest natural antivirals, and kids just love the taste. Honestly I do too! You should try to give it as soon as you suspect your child might have any type of virus. I cannot tell you how many times I have taken elderberry just when I feel the slightest pain in my throat, and many times you feel much better literally overnight. Next, I put three to four drops of garlic and mullein oil in my child's ear a couple times a day. You can buy a liquid preparation at most health food stores or make your own. Garlic is antibacterial and acts as a natural antibiotic to work on getting rid of the infection. It has antiviral properties too. I will also rub frankincense essential oil all around the outside of the ear and on the bottom of my children's feet to promote their immune system to work better. If you do not see the ear infection getting better rather quickly, then you will have to call your practitioner for oral antibiotics whether they are prescription or a natural antibiotic.

Ear Wax: There have been many times when I thought my son had an ear infection and it turned out to be pain from a build-up of ear wax. I have unfortunately found this out the hard way. There was one specific time that I treated him for an ear infection for days that would not go away, so I took him to an ENT who found a very large build-up of wax. And unfortunately this did keep occurring, so I began to treat it at home by taking 3 percent hydrogen peroxide (the kind you get at the drug store) mixed with equal parts distilled water. Then I use a medicine dropper to put some in his ear. I usually lie him on his side and do several droppers in that ear before moving on to the next one. Keep in mind that they will squirm, not from pain but the wax makes a crackling sound while it's breaking up inside the ear. The good news is that they usually feel relief immediately afterwards. Even my husband asks me to do it to him a couple times a year. He was the one who explained exactly what it feels like and that it's a pretty loud sound while it's crackling in your ear. The wax will usually just float up where you can wipe it with a tissue to remove it. You can also use the garlic and mullein drops for this as well. The oil will slowly help dissolve the wax.

Cough: Again I will use liquid elderberry at the first sign of cold, this way we can nip it in the bud many times before it progresses into other symptoms, such as a cough. Once I start hearing my children cough then I immediately add raw or manuka honey. Any type of good quality honey will coat the throat and help you stop coughing as well as kill the bacteria in your throat. I normally give them ½ to 1 teaspoon at least twice a day with the last dosage being right before bedtime. This way they are comfortable for most of the evening. Manuka honey is much more medicinal than regular raw honey and you want to buy one with at least a level of 15 or higher. I use manuka honey for so many things. Your child might resist a little in the beginning, since it tastes stronger than regular honey and definitely not as sweet. Just stay with it and keep explaining how this is going to make them feel so much better. My daughter was extremely resistant to the taste and even used to gag, but now she requests it when she has a cough or sore throat since she knows how well it works.

Stuffy Nose: This is an extremely annoying symptom for most people, but for me it's much worse given my deviated septum. I find it difficult to function well when I have to breathe through my mouth all day and night. So I have had to find something that works—and I did. I drink peppermint tea when my nose is stuffed up and it usually clears in ten minutes. Although there have been times that I am experiencing an allergic reaction to something and I need something stronger. That's when I either brush my teeth with peppermint essential oil or rub it in my hand, and cup my nose, so I can breathe in the vapors and clear my nasal passages. Now if your nose is stuffy from seasonal allergies and not a cold, then you might want to look into an herbal supplement that can provide a more long term solution for the season such as quercetin, stinging nettle or butterbur. For a child, you can diffuse a few drops of peppermint essential oil in water into the air or rub the oil in your own hands so they can inhale it.

Sore Throat: I deal with sore throats very often given my son has been diagnosed with PANDAS and gets strep throat all the time. For him, I will give the natural herb Berberine preventatively each day during the wintertime, since it does not allow the strep bacteria to adhere to the epithelial cells in the throat. But for your average run of the mill sore throat that normally accompanies a cold, I just give both liquid elderberry and manuka honey twice a day. Similar to a cough, make sure to give the second dose of manuka honey right before bed so that it stays there overnight, coating the throat and fighting the bacteria. Many times I will add an herb to stimulate the immune system such as olive leaf extract or astralagus.

Strep Throat: Most people are not confident to treat strep throat by themselves, and this is totally understandable. I happen to have no problem for the simple reason that my son would be on antibiotics constantly if I did not find another way. The antibiotics would wreak havoc on his gut, which I am continually trying to repair. For those of you who are interested, I give Dylan berberine twice a day at a higher dose than when I am supplementing with it preventatively. I also use manuka honey, since it also has the ability to kill some strep and keep him comfortable. There are other natural antibiotics that you can use such as colloidal silver. Many qualified practitioners can help you find the right treatment if you would like to avoid standard antibiotics, however it is important to work with someone who is well versed in natural medicine if you decide to go that route.

Pink Eye: Many people think that they need to run to the pediatrician to get those antibiotic eye drops at the first glance of a red eye. This is another instance where the condition many times is caused by a virus and would probably go away on its own even if you did nothing. I always do salt water rinses with a homemade saline recipe that is the same PH as your tears. The salt is antibacterial and will heal and keep the condition from getting worse. The homemade saline recipe that I use is a ¼ teaspoon of sea salt with a half a cup of distilled water. It is very important that the water is distilled and free from contaminants. You also need to make sure that all the utensils, cup, and dropper are very clean before using, so that you do not introduce any new bacteria into the eye. I usually do three to four saline rinses a day and give liquid elderberry for the viral component. Now if you get to treating the eye too late or it progresses quickly and they start to develop pus or conjunctivitis, it would be best to go see your pediatrician immediately to get the eye looked at. You always need to be very careful when it comes to the eyes, since they are quite sensitive and delicate. And if you are not quite sure whether it is pink eye or not then it's best to bring your child to the doctor to at least get a diagnosis.

Foot Fungus: Athlete's foot is a condition that my daughter seems to pick up often when she is playing in those children's gyms without socks. Now I buy girls yoga socks with grips so she does not have to walk around them barefoot anymore. However I have had to treat those painful cracks on the bottoms of her toes more than once. I have found an extremely easy and effective solution, so I do not have to buy those over the counter creams that have god knows what kinds of chemicals in them. I simply buy a bottle of Bragg's Raw Apple Cider Vinegar and douse the bottom of her feet with it using a cotton ball right before she goes to bed and then place socks on. She doesn't love the smell of the vinegar, hence the reason for the socks to cover it. I find that I only need to do this bedtime ritual for about one week and then you can usually see the cracks and redness slowly heal. The raw apple cider vinegar creates an alkaline environment in which the fungus just cannot survive. You could not find a more natural treatment than this and there are many other uses for raw apple cider vinegar.

Urinary Tract Infection: For years, I treated frequent and painful urinary tract infections with antibiotics that would further destroy the flora in my gut until one functional medicine practitioner suggested using Uva Ursi. This was actually a suggestion by Dr. O'Hara's partner who treats adults in her office. I did some research on this natural herb and discovered it's been used for hundreds of years. It is actually what people used before antibiotics. And what's even more amazing is that it takes the pain away in much less time than your common antibiotic, which I find takes at least a day or two to lower the discomfort from the infection. When I take Uva Ursi the pain is gone in about eight to ten hours. You do have to be careful not to stay on it more than ten to fourteen days. I would also suggest getting the correct dosage and using it under the care of a practitioner, especially for a child. I have successfully used this treatment for my daughter, not only for a urinary tract infection but to treat her gut dysbiosis as well.

Fever: I have a rule of thumb that I do not treat a fever with medication unless it passes a certain threshold. The magic number for me when I will treat with Motrin or ibuprofen is around 103 unless they seem very uncomfortable at a lower temperature with a horrible headache or some other painful symptom. I think it's important to let the body try to heal itself. A fever is a response that the body creates to fight something off. One thing you should try never to give in response to a fever or anything for that matter is Tylenol. The reason is that it depletes glutathione, which as we've discussed is a very important antioxidant that helps the body get rid of toxic things. It's even more important to have a good supply of glutathione in your body when you are under the weather. Many of us moms who utilize holistic medicine cannot understand why pediatricians still tell people to give their child Tylenol after vaccines. It is the worst thing you could possibly do. When my kids get a fever, I make sure to give them plenty of fluids, including coconut water for the electrolytes. It's like a natural version of PediaSure. We usually make my daughter a huge pot of chicken soup with many garlic cloves in it, since it has strong antiviral properties and helps her stay hydrated. There are also so many natural supplements that you can give to support the immune system during the fever. Here are some to name a few: vitamin D, vitamin C, cod liver oil, echinacea, goldenseal, elderberry, manuka honey, astralagus, and olive leaf extract. Another wonderful thing I do when they are sick is to rub a couple drops of frankincense essential oil on the bottoms of each of their feet to stimulate their immune systems. I would never suggest letting a fever play out if it is accompanied by other symptoms such as vomiting, diarrhea, or a stiff neck. Again, always check with your child's doctor if you are not sure what you are dealing with, since playing it safe is always the best bet. Another great remedy for those who like essential oils is peppermint oil. Just rub a couple drops on the bottom of their feet every couple hours or so. You will be surprised how quickly it helps the fever break.

Splinters: This is one of the most painful conditions, which I have tons of experience with. We rent a house out east every summer and both my kids inevitably rack up many splinters throughout our month-long stay. At first, I used to try to tweeze them, which caused an immense amount of both pain and trauma for all involved. Then one day I discovered someone posted about using manuka honey as a natural treatment for splinters. Being that this is one of my favorite substances, I was more than willingly to give it a try and experienced immediate success. All you have to do is put a glob of it on the splinter right before bed, place a band-aid over it, and then when you wake up in the morning the splinter will be at, or very close to, the surface. Many times you can just almost wipe it off or take a tweezer and you barely need to pull on it. For very deep splinters it may take two nights. This remedy has made my life so easy in the summertime, and we have no more drama or trauma!

Cuts on the Skin: Now for simple cuts and abrasions, I also use manuka honey. It contains potent antibacterial components, which perform just as well as any store-bought cream in a tube, such as bacitracin. I like to use the essential oil frankincense when there is a lot of redness surrounding the cut. Frankincense is a strong anti-inflammatory, and it also stimulates the immune system to work harder. Another trick I use is to clean the cut out thoroughly multiple times a day with a mix of "brown and bubbly." I learned this technique from one of Dr. Russell Blaylock's books and newsletters. You take hydrogen peroxide and pour it on the cut and then add Betadine over it. You repeat this process of adding both these items on the cut a few times in a row approximately three to four times a day. It's amazing that you can see an infection heal very quickly with just the hydrogen peroxide and Betadine rinses.

Pain in Back (or Other Body Parts): My husband has a few chronic injuries that produce quite a bit of pain at times, so I have had to research natural remedies for pain relief. I like to use tart cherry extract and ginger for inflammation. You can take tart cherry in a juice or capsule form. As far as the ginger, I like to make a quart of homemade tea where I peel and cut up three to four large pieces of ginger root and simmer it in water for about thirty minutes. Both these items can be used instead of ibuprofen, or in addition to, depending on the amount of pain. Ginger also comes in a capsule as well. Many times, I also apply essential oils topically. There are many that work, but I often use frankincense and peppermint. I just apply a few drops on the painful area and rub it in three to four times a day. And just like an over-the-counter pain reliever, you will notice the pain dissipate within a half hour of applying it and then it slowly resurfaces after a few hours when it's time to reapply again. And unlike over-the-counter pain relievers, essential oils can be applied much more often and provide other health benefits aside from the pain relief.

Headache: This is one condition I have had more than my fair share of experience with. My son started getting headaches in his left eye a few years ago and nobody could figure out why he was having them. They still occur and we believe it might be related to his PANDAS conditions. His eyes will hurt when he has some of the other symptoms of PANDAS such as increased OCD, decreased appetite, easily agitated, and so on. There are many instances that I have no choice but to give him ibuprofen. For this reason, I have it compounded so it is in the purest form without all the other junk they put in an over-the-counter pharmaceutical product, including that horrible dye on the hard outer shell. Any doctor can call in a prescription into a compounding pharmacy to have it made. My son does not take capsules, so I just empty the white powder into a teaspoon of applesauce, mix it up, and give it to him. I also give him tart cherry, which is a natural anti-inflammatory, and it relives pain caused by inflammation. Essential oils are another wonderful treatment that work pretty quickly. You can try different ones to see which work best for you. I like to use lavender, a blend called Copaiba (by Young Living), peppermint (dilute this one with a carrier oil), and frankincense. You can rub a couple drops on the forehead right under the hairline or on the back of the neck as well. Just be careful to keep it out of your eyes.

Eczema: Both my children displayed the symptoms of eczema. For my son, the eczema came very early on and was short-lived, since his body moved on to bigger autoimmune issues. My daughter Jessica had eczema for a much longer period of time and I did finally get rid of it naturally. We never filled the steroid prescription cream that I was given by the dermatologist, and quite honestly I never even considered it. Why would I give her a cream that would never get to the root of the problem, and the cream has side effects that it can thin the skin and it only works while you stay on it? The moment you stop, many times it comes right back. This made absolutely no sense to me.

I personally don't view this condition as a minor ailment, however I included it in this section since it is so common and I wanted to give you a safe alternative to the steroel cream. Secondly I thought it was important to point out that this is sometimes one of the first signs that your child's immune system is imbalanced. It may also be a sign that there are undiagnosed food allergies, gut dysbiosis or leaky gut. Eczema is normally a result of inflammation in the gut, and many times the inflammation is coming from germs or food allergies. When I first started to read up on eczema, it was pretty apparent to me that many times it was caused by an egg allergy. She was eating egg each day in some form, since egg was one of the ingredients in all the bread we baked. We had already taken out gluten, dairy, and nuts, so next out went the eggs. The eczema did not disappear immediately, as I hoped it would. I realized that I was going to have to attack what might be going on in her gut. I tried many different natural supplements with her, but there were two that stood out as the ones that did the job.

I gave her Uva Ursi, which is a natural antimicrobial that killed the bad bacteria and yeast in her gut. Please remember that I mentioned in the urinary tract infection page that you can only give this for ten to fourteen days at a time and then you must take a break for at least two weeks before using it to treat again. It is best to work with a qualified practitioner, especially with herbs that you have not used before. Next I gave her aloe juice for the inflammation that the food allergies and bad germs may be producing. A nice side effect is that it relieved her constipation. Aloe is an adaptogen, which means that it will take care of whatever symptom the body is producing to bring it back into balance. The aloe will also act as an antimicrobial that kills bad bacteria and parasites. You do need to be careful and get the right dose from a practitioner. I used both these supplements on and off for about six months and I am happy to report the eczema has never come back.

Yeast: I believe that yeast is one of the bad germs in Jessica's gut that was driving her eczema. We did do some stool tests, which indicated that yeast was present and she had a bloated belly confirming that there was probably gut dysbiosis. This was not a surprise to me given my own history of yeast and fungal issues. Dylan also suffered from a relentless yeast rash around his penis as an infant. Back then, I only knew to give him what the doctor told me which was some form of a prescription cream. The rash looked like it went away when I used the cream, however the cause of the problem continued to fester and grow just like my own issues. An overgrowth of yeast creates an imbalance in the gut, which can throw your entire immune system off balance. This in turn can affect the whole body. Many practitioners think that gut dysbiosis leads to leaky gut and can result in any number of autoimmune illnesses. I believe this to be true as well. The integrity of your gut is one of the most important things you have in this world. It is what protects and keeps you healthy. You need to treat it well so that it has the ability to take care of your body. This means not throwing a ton of processed foods with chemicals and preservatives in it. These are toxins to your body, which will wear your gut down over time. There are so many wonderful natural herbal supplements that you can take to improve your gut health. Here is a list of my favorites: garlic, ginger, olive leaf extract, astralagus, turmeric, oregano oil, banderol, samento, cat's claw, and berberine. Again I would always check with your practitioner before using them for the first time, since some of them are quite powerful.

Parasites: There are many natural substances that take care of parasites including food, such as garlic, coconut oil, pomegranate, and aloe juice. When Dylan was a toddler, we used homotoxicolgy, since it seemed to be very gentle. Sure enough, we noticed them in his stool once they were killed. I personally like to take black walnut at least once a year as it gets rid of so many different types of parasites. I feel great on this supplement, not sure if it is killing the yeast or parasite or possibly both. It used to be thought that only people in third world countries get parasites, but we know that isn't true. They are on all of our produce and in our pets, which means we are exposed all the time. When the body is healthy it can live symbiotically with them and get rid of them on its own. However, when the gut is imbalanced it is vulnerable to an opportunistic infection. It's important to try to crowd out the bad germs with good bacteria from fermented foods and probiotics. It is hard for yeast and parasites to live in an alkaline environment, so a lot of thought should be paid to taking certain things each day that can create a more alkaline PH in the gut such as apple cider vinegar, lemon in water, and baking soda. You can take each of these items separately or mix them in a glass of water and simply drink it.

Tooth or Gum Infection: My husband and I experience this condition from time to time, which is why I have had to become an expert. Unfortunately, we both had the same dentist, who used to leave a space between our teeth when she filled a cavity, and now food gets caught. So we both experience a tooth or gum infection at least once a year. I use multiple treatments simultaneously, which always include saltwater rinses at least a few times a day. I normally make a huge vat of homemade ginger tea and drink two cups a day for its natural antibiotic properties. I brush my teeth with Thieves essential oil as well as make a mouth wash to use several times a day. I place clove essential oil directly on the area for pain relief. It is an all-natural analgesic that many holistic dentists will apply to your gum for pain relief when you get your teeth cleaned. Another thing I do that stops the infection for me dead in its tracks is when I slice up a clove of garlic really thin and take a couple of these slices, wrap it in gauze and place it directly on the infection. I usually leave it on for at least forty minutes and I notice the infection is gone the next day. Please be warned that many people will get a canker sore from the garlic, myself included, but I find it's better than the infection. You can also take an herbal supplement orally to use as a natural antibiotic. My husband likes to put a drop of oregano essential oil in an empty capsule and swallow it. This is a very strong herb and not everyone can tolerate it. A lot of people keep it in the house just in case someone in the family experiences food poisoning, since it's that powerful. Obviously, if the infection does not go away in a few days then you should consult your dentist or physician.

PERSONAL CARE PRODUCTS

This is another area that I am very passionate about. It is so easy to buy wonderful safe products as well as make them yourself. I find myself doing both. There will be a section at the end of the book called "products I love" where you will find a list of some of the ones that I have tried and really appreciate.

Tooth or Gum Prevention: I do not remember the last time I used a normal looking tube of toothpaste. My oral care has gone through a slow metamorphosis beginning with Colgate toothpaste fifteen years ago. Next I tried the natural toothpastes from the health food store, and now I use herbs and essential oils. My children simply brush their teeth with sea salt some nights and a wonderful tooth powder that has kaolin clay and baking soda in it. You can make your own toothpaste recipe or put a drop of essential oil on your toothbrush. I enjoy brushing my teeth with peppermint essential oil, since you get a nice fresh taste and it's antibacterial. Essential oils are very powerful and you only need one drop if you are putting it directly on your toothbrush. For my children, I will dilute the essential oil with a teaspoon of coconut oil. We also use prepared liquid and powder tooth treatments that have specific herbs for tightening your gums and treating the bacteria in your mouth. They work really well and I would never go back to using a run-of-the-mill tube of toothpaste ever again. Another wonderful thing we do for oral care and overall health is oil pull. This comes from Ayurvedic medicine and has been used for hundreds of years. It can help so many health conditions, it's astounding. All you do is take a teaspoon of an oil of your choice and swish it around in your mouth for approximately twenty minutes. You have to make sure to spit out all the oil and never swallow any of it. The oil pulling technique will draw toxins out of your teeth and gums. You should immediately rinse your mouth with warm water a couple times after you have disposed of the oil. Many people like to use coconut oil given its antibacterial properties.

I think the most important thing to remember is that your mouth is the first entrance to your microbiome, since it's one long tube that is connected from your mouth down your esophagus, into the stomach, through the intestines ending with your colon. The whole digestive tract needs your care and attention and it begins in your mouth. This is the reason that oral care is so important. I hear many stories where someone is very affected by an autoimmune such as rheumatoid arthritis and they do many natural interventions that help only to a certain point. The last piece usually entails meticulously combing through the inventory of metals and root canals in their mouth to extract some of them. It's important to remember that removing these root canals or amalgam fillings must be done by a qualified holistic dentist who has a lot of knowledge and expertise in order to protect one's health from further damage. Many times an individual's health will improve dramatically once those toxic teeth and heavy metals are taken out. In Chinese medicine there are tooth meridian charts that connect certain organs to specific teeth in your mouth. Many people believe that cancer can develop in a body part, which is connected to the tooth with a root canal. I personally removed two teeth that had root canals and felt a huge improvement in my own health. Implants are another thing that can cause issues for people, since many are made from titanium or some other metal. I just think you need to be thoughtful about putting any inanimate objects into your body on a permanent basis, since the body can react to anything foreign it thinks should not be there.

Soap: Let's talk about soap, since we all use it every day. All soap is certainly not the same and some can even be harmful. We have all heard that using antibacterial soap is not good for a couple reasons. First it creates antibiotic-resistant bacteria, which is becoming a growing problem, especially in hospitals. The chemicals that make the soap antibacterial are thought to be dangerous to your health and the environment as they get washed down the sink. Your best bet is to use warm water and regular soap that does not contain harmful chemicals or ingredients. Many people believe that if it's on your skin it doesn't get into your body, however this could not be further from the truth. How would a nicotine patch work if this were the case. The skin is there to protect our inner body parts, however it is extremely porous and needs to be protected from exposures especially to toxins.

Another area of concern is that we are washing our skin too often and removing the good bacteria, which naturally covers our skin. This balance of good and bad bacteria is equally imperative on our skin as it is in our guts. It is up to the individual, but sometimes it's best not to shower if you are not dirty. Many women do not wash their hair everyday, since they like the way it looks with the natural oils. Well the same goes for our skin that you can strip it of the essential bacteria and oils that help keep it looking healthy. This of course is a preference that you will have to decide for yourself. I personally do not shower every day and only wash my hair about every three days. It's just what feels comfortable and right for me. I use very natural soaps that actually list the ingredients on the package. You could probably even eat most of my soaps as they contain only natural oils such as olive or coconut.

Sunscreen: This is another big area of concern given there are so many dangerous products on the market these days. How many times have you been sitting at a beach and someone is spraying themselves or their child with those noxious chemical sunscreen aerosols, and then the wind blows it towards you giving you no choice but to breathe it in. This is actually a big pet peeve of my mind, since it's kind of like secondhand smoke. And to make matters worse some of these sunscreens contain nanoparticles that can be very dangerous, especially when inhaled into the lungs. It's also possible that over time they can accumulate in your organs. Many functional medicine practitioners think that the increase in skin cancer actually has to do with all the chemicals that are in the sunscreens. Some of the chemicals in them can damage the DNA in your skin, which can actually result in mutations in your skin cells. So it's incredibly important to use a very safe sunscreen. The Environmental Working Group is a wonderful resource that rates many products for safety including sunscreens. Here is their website: www.ewg.org You can also make very simple homemade formulas. My husband loves one recipe in particular that I used to make for him that contained two parts organic coconut oil to one part zinc oxide. He liked the smell, and it made his skin feel really moisturized.

Mouthwash: Is there a single person out there that doesn't want fresh breath? I can't imagine it! One thing to keep in mind is that if you experience chronic bad breath, you may have issues in your gut. However, if you just want fresher breath then you have a couple choices, such as to buy a healthy version of mouthwash or make it yourself. I like to take a cup of mineral water and add drops of essential oils. Sometimes I use tea tree (this one should not be swallowed) and peppermint or Thieves. It depends if I need the mouthwash to clean my mouth or treat a gum or tooth infection. You can experiment with different oils, but please make sure they are food grade and one-hundred-percent pure.

There is no reason to use your store-bought brand of mouthwash that comes with chemicals that may damage your microbiome. Remember everything that goes in your mouth has an effect on the rest of the body!

Makeup: This is an area that I have begun to spend a bit of time investigating. Most women know that they ingest their lip product every single day, since it is on before you sit down to eat and then we must reapply it afterwards. For this reason, it is so important to purchase one that is as natural as possible. Stories have circulated for years about lead being found in many well-known brand lipsticks, yet another reason you need to buy from a very responsible and reputable natural cosmetics company. I have a very significant gluten allergy and must get a product that is gluten-free. The good news is that due to consumer demand, so many more natural cosmetic companies exist, making it quite easy with the click of a mouse to find them. I have included some of the ones I appreciate in the "Products I Love" section towards the back of the book.

So we have already covered the points that what you put on your skin is absorbed and the substances that go in your mouth make it down to your gut. This is why you should look at makeup the same way you do food and other personal care products. It must be made from the highest quality ingredients without harmful chemicals, additives, and preservatives. I know this process of changing over your personal care products might feel overwhelming, but don't feel like you have to do it all at once. Just try to change one product at a time and over the course of a year you will have replaced many. This is how I approached it for my family, and it has not been such a stressful experience. I am also happy to support those companies that strive to make a difference in both the environment and people's health. I can't thank them enough for the healthy products they make available.

As you can tell, I am extremely passionate about all the subjects intertwined in this book and holistic health in general. However I am especially excited to share with you some of my favorite natural supplements that I use regularly and rely on to keep my family's health in balance. To review, I have compiled a list of my top twenty favorites that can normally be seen residing in my large medicine cabinet just waiting for someone to need them. Please keep in mind that some of these are actually food, but I view them as natural supplements to cure particular ailments. Many of these natural substances can be used for multiple symptoms and complaints as well as in combination with each other. Some of these I have already specifically mentioned earlier in this chapter in reference to one of the ailments that we covered.

I view these items to be very safe, but that isn't to say that someone could not have an allergic reaction or negative response to one of them. For that reason, you should always consult your practitioner to see if they think a particular natural supplement would be right for you or your child to try.

NATURAL SUPPLEMENTS THAT I LOVE:
(IN ALPHABETICAL ORDER)

Aloe Juice	Elderberry	Oregano Oil
Apple Cider Vinegar	Garlic	Tart Cherry
Ashwaghanda	Ginger	Tumeric
Banderol	Frankincense	Uva Ursi
Berberine	Manuka Honey	Vitamin C
B12	Milk Thistle	Vitamin D
Cat's Claw	Olive Leaf Extract	Vitamin E

My family has taken many of the supplements that I have mentioned above either on a regular basis or from time to time. I am always researching and trying new ones out as well. My medicine cabinet is extremely large and does not reside in my bathroom like the traditional ones. It is actually a custom-made closet in my dining room. I am proud to say that it does contain some pretty obscure supplements, as well as the ones I consider to be quite basic.

The basic supplements are ones that we take every day or rotate on a regular basis. Rotating supplements that you really like helps them work better by not allowing your body to get too used to them and build up a resistance. For example, I might take Ashwaghanda for a period of time and then replace it with cat's claw. Then there are certain supplements that I feel most people should take every day with some exceptions. Here is my short list of what I consider to be bare bones or staples: vitamin D, probiotics, and fish oil. Most people except for those who spend enormous amount of time outdoors are deficient in vitamin D. One reason is that people in general spend a good amount of their day indoors and when they do go outside, sunscreen is applied. Another exception would be if a person eats quite a bit of fermented food throughout the day, then they might not need a probiotic. Many cultures serve fermented foods with every meal they consume, since it is an integral part of their culinary traditions.

You can treat symptoms with natural medicine rather than always relying on pharmaceutical intervention. Many of these herbs and natural substances have been around and used to treat illness for hundreds of years. My goal was to inspire you to consider trying some of these natural treatments for minor everyday ailments. I hope some of you take to it and begin your own journey using natural medicine on a regular basis. There are many qualified practitioners that use natural medicine in their practice including all of the ones that you have heard from throughout this book. Their contact information is listed in the back of the book.

When the body is primarily in a healthy state you will only need to deal with these minor everyday ailments. Here is one of my favorite quotes that pretty much sums up my feelings on all of this:

"Let food be thy medicine and medicine be thy food."

—Hippocrates

Chapter 15

WRAP UP

I am so grateful to have been given the chance to share my journey and every-thing that I have learned along the way to help you try to prevent autism. My only request is that you think of the brave children and families from time to time that have suffered immensely to bring you these incredibly important facts. This includes my beautiful son Dylan too. I wish each one of you could look into his big beautiful blue eyes and see his enormous smile that he puts on display every day despite his huge challenges and obstacles.

As I come to close this book I want to share a recent experience with you. Please know that I tell you particularly upsetting events only to drive a point home and not to disturb you for no reason.

My family spends each of our summers out east, including this one where I am finishing up writing the book. I have been lucky enough to find a very nurturing and understanding camp in Montauk that allows my son to go accompanied by a shadow (special teacher or therapist). He normally does so well with this break from the everyday grind and constant therapy. Luckily for us we do not see any kind of regression during this time away. I think my son really looks forward to it every year and I believe he even senses as it is getting close. The reason I think he appreciates it so much is that he gets to act like a regular kid that goes swimming all day and does fun activities outside. The therapy that he works so hard at gets pushed aside for a nice chunk of time. I am not sure who likes it more, him or me. As a parent, I work many months in advance to pull all the pieces together to make it happen. I put ads in several different listings to get qualified people to apply for my shadow position. We normally hire a special education teacher or speech pathologist, and we have to pay a pretty penny for it on top of the camp. My husband and I never begrudge spending this money, since he deserves it and so do we. My son gets to act like a typical kid without a care in the world. This year we were lucky enough to get a wonderful psychologist with a PhD who has many years experience working with children on the spectrum.

My son went to camp with her for the first week and had the best time. The directors remarked how well he was doing this year and that he had made so many improvements from the previous summer. Most people first notice how happy and affectionate Dylan can be. Well unfortunately this time of his life only lasted one week, since he was displaying all the symptoms of a bad PANDAS attack which can include aggression, eye pain, increased OCD, and motor tics to name a few. The biggest problem for the camp was the aggression towards other children and his counselors. This is the first time we had this problem at a summer camp. Unfortunately, it can come on suddenly and literally change his personality overnight, which it did in this case. We had noticed the symptoms creeping up on us over the weekend and by the start of the second week he was no longer our happy child. My husband and I were beside ourselves after hearing that he was having problems at the camp and really acting out. We were left with no choice but to pull him out of the camp for the rest of the summer. It may be hard for many of you without a special needs child to understand how devastating this can be for a parent. It's like someone ties your hands and feet behind your back and puts a muzzle over your mouth. You are absolutely helpless and can't stop what is happening to your child. I can't even imagine for one moment how he must feel when something takes over his body like this and causes him so much intense pain and discomfort. In some ways I wish I could experience it for him or even just for one day so I would know exactly what to do to help him.

The purpose in telling you this story is that this is just one little thing I go through all the time. You cannot imagine how many more things there are like this—on a daily basis. I will name a few only so you can get a good picture of how devastating it is to raise a child with autism. My son has no "real" friends, and by this I mean people he can have an ongoing relationship with. It is still very difficult for him to carry on a normal conversation. He can have ones that involve him more or less answering yes or no questions. Dylan has the language but lacks the skills to connect on a level besides his own needs or wants.

What is so sad is that he is very intelligent and understands everything anyone says and always has. When my son is sick I usually find out once the pain has gotten so great that his behavior makes it obvious that something is terribly wrong. And I am very attuned to him, but he has a pretty high threshold for pain, like many children on the spectrum. It's devastating at those times for me to realize that he has probably been in pain for so long. I don't know what it is about his illness that keeps him from trying to tell me. He can say the words, "Mommy my head hurts" but doesn't. It's equally hard for my husband and I to watch my daughter get sad at times when Dylan won't play with her; or the more appropriate description is that he can't. I know this has an effect on her and I feel sad about it at times. There are hundreds of memories I have of playing with my brother who was just a few years older than me. My kids are both missing out. And we miss out as a family on a lot of things too. My husband and I turn down a lot of invites for things that we know Dylan would not do well in that particular situation, or he is not doing well enough at the time. This includes barbecues, dinner at certain restaurants and vacations. My daughter also misses out on those invites too!

This is the reason that it was very easy for me to jump through as many hoops as possible to try to prevent this from happening to my daughter. As I mentioned earlier, there is nothing that you could ever tell me to do that would be too inconvenient to prevent autism. There is nothing harder to me than autism. The pain many of us parents feel is more about what our child has to go through and what they are missing, not necessarily our own experiences. I am forty-five years old and have lived a whole life full of friends, fun, and relationships before autism struck. My son only lived eighteen months before it started. And my daughter has never known a life without autism.

So I can honestly tell you that you won't ever regret any time you spend trying to prevent it, but you may regret the things that you don't do. It's much worse to know something and not do it than not to have that information at the time. I of course did not have the information at the time. My only regret was not listening harder to that little voice inside me that knew vaccines were not a good thing for Dylan. Please don't make my same mistake! I will always regret that I cannot undo those vaccines and especially the one that caused an ischemic stroke that damaged my little boy's brain. I live with the what ifs every so often wondering what it would be like. Would he be interested in girls right now? I know that they would be interested in him, since he is so incredibly handsome. Would he be playing the guitar or be a jock? What would he be doing with the majority of his time if it did not have to be spent on doing treatments to try to fix his autism. What would life be like without autism?

I don't want you to find out what any of this feels like. Please do everything you can in your power to prevent autism. You will also be preventing all the other childhood chronic illnesses such as diabetes and asthma. Right now I would trade either of those for autism, since I feel like he could at least be functional, go to school, and have friends. But in reality I don't want those either.

This is why I work so hard to keep my typical daughter healthy. I want her to have the childhood she deserves, the childhood Dylan deserved but never got, one without sickness and pain.

So remember to eat food that is as pure as possible and don't beat yourself up for what you have not already done. I will say it again, TOMORROW IS A NEW DAY! Make the best choices that you can going forward for you and your family and try not to look back so often. And remember every choice you make counts!

I want to thank all the exceptional contributors and mothers who generously gave of their time for this important project. In order of appearance:

Sid Baker, MD
Nancy O'Hara, MD
Geri Brewster RDN MPH CDN
Maureen McDonnell RN
Scott Smith PA
Anju Usman, MD
Jack Lyons-Weiler PhD
Stephanie Senneff PhD
Corinne Simpson Brown
Katie Wright
Maria Rickert Hong CHHC, AADP

I am also beyond grateful to all the parents who came before me that tried the treatments, which are now considered the standard in biomedical protocols for children with autism. Without your bravery, I may not have been inspired to fight as hard on my own journey. Thank you for showing your perseverance and determination that ultimately fed mine.

The person I want to thank the most is the one that inspired this book and continues to open my eyes and teach me new things every day. He is my courageous son Dylan. You are the most genuine person I will ever meet. My love for you is unbending. And my pursuit for your recovery is relentless and unstoppable, for you deserve the world.

A LETTER TO MY SON

Dear Dylan,

I love you with all my heart. Nothing has made me happier in life than the opportunity to be your mom.

Words could never describe how proud I am of you. Life has not been easy, but you have handled it with such grace. Somehow you have been able to find so much beauty in the world and helped me to see it too.

Your childhood has been overshadowed with a difficult and complicated illness. I am deeply sorry for the things that you have missed out on. Please know that I have noticed your cries and emotions at those times, even when you didn't have the words to tell me. You have handled more as a child than most adults will ever have to.

I know that I have never met a more courageous person than you. Our journey through the tough times and the healing has inspired me to share your legacy in the hopes of preventing the same thing from happening to other children.

Please know that you have already saved so many kids from suffering the same fate, since I continue to share your story. My hope is that this book will continue those efforts on a larger scale and that together we will prevent suffering in countless other families for years to come.

We have taken all your lemons and made the most beautiful batch of lemonade.

Your suffering has not been in vain.

You are an amazing person and I know you will do great things in life. You already have! People are touched and inspired by you everyday, especially me.

Love,
Mom

PRODUCTS I LOVE

Gluten-Free Sourdough Bread www.glutenfreesourdough.com
I order gluten-free sourdough bread mixes from this site on an ongoing basis. Sharon also makes a lot of products that are already cooked and ready to eat!

Primal Life Organics www.primallifeorganics.com
This is a wonderful site that makes products to order that are produced with the most natural ingredients. I really enjoy the natural deodorant and tooth powder.

Sudsy Soapcakes http://sudsysoapcakes.com
The soaps this company makes are allergy friendly and made from very few healthy ingredients. I purchase the plain olive oil soap quite often and take advantage of their offer to purchase six bars of soap and get the seventh free.

Young Living Essential Oils www.youngliving.com
I purchase many of my essential oils from Young Living. They are very pure which is the most important thing when it comes to this type of product.

Lifefactory www.lifefactory.com
This is a great company that sells all kinds of safe glass bottles, cups, and food storage containers. My kids use these items every single day. They also make baby bottles.

100 Percent Pure www.100percentpure.com
You can find some of the nicest personal care products including makeup made from simple natural ingredients with lots of fruit pigments. I really enjoy their shampoo and conditioner as well.

RevitaPOP Methyl B-12 Lollipops www.revitapop.com
These are wonderful tasting lollipops that give your children a much needed dose of B12. They are organic, gluten- and casein-free, as well as vegan. My daughter absolutely loves them and I get to feel a little less guilty giving her a treat.

ADDITIONAL RESOURCES:

Newsletters to sign up for

Blaylock	https://w3.blaylockwellness.com
Sherry Rogers	https://prestigepublishing.com
Natural News	http://www.naturalnews.com
GreenMed	http://www.greenmedinfo.com
Living Traditionally	http://livingtraditionally.com

Facebook pages with good health posts

Just Eat Real Food

David Wolfe

Dr. Josh Axe

Traditional Cooking School by Gnowfglins

Mommypotamus

Real Farmacy

Books to Read

Almost Autism by Maria Rickert Hong

Breaking the Vicious Cycle by Elaine Gottschall

Cure Tooth Decay by Ramiel Nagel

Gentle Birth Choices by Barbara Harper and Suzanne Arms

Grain-Free Gourmet by Jenny Lass and Jodi Bager

Healing with Whole Foods by Paul Pitchfork

Herbal Antibiotics by Stephen Harrod Buhner

*The Nourishing Traditions Book of Baby & Child Care by Sally Fallon
Morell and Thomas S. Cowan*

Nutritional Herbology by Mark Pedersen

Whole Body Dentistry by Mark A. Breiner

Websites with great information

http://wellnessmama.com

www.draxe.com

www.sokhop.com

CONTRIBUTORS LIST:

In alphabetical order

Sid Baker, MD
ASKDOCTORBAKER.com

Geri Brewster, RD, MPH, CDN, PC
Registered Dietitian-Nutritionist in Integrative and Functional Medicine
In Westchester and in New York City by Appointment:
491 Lexington Avenue
Mount Kisco, NY 10549
(914) 864-1976 Office
GERIBREWSTER.COM
https://www.facebook.com/GeriBrewsterNutrition
https://twitter.com/dietstuff
http://geribrewster.com/ordering

Founder of Build Your Best Bump by Somavance LLC
BUILDYOURBESTBUMP.COM
(914) 236-4374
https://www.facebook.com/BuildYourBestBump
https://twitter.com/yourbestbump

Nancy Hofreuter O'Hara, MD, MPH, FAAP
Center for Integrative Health
www.ihealthnow.org

Maria Rickert Hong, Certified Holistic Health Counselor, AADP
www.MariaRickertHong.com
Author of *Almost Autism: Recovering Children from Sensory Processing Disorder,
A Reference for Parents and Practitioners*
Media Director and Board Member, Epidemic Answers

Maureen McDonnell, BS, RN
Health Education Services, Inc
Weaverville, NC 28787
MauraHealth@aol.com
Saving Our Kids, Healing Our Planet SOKHOP.com
(609) 240-1315

Stephanie Seneff, PhD
MIT CSAIL
URL: http://people.csail.mit.edu/seneff

Scott M. Smith, PA
Central Florida Functional Medicine
1395 N. Courtenay Parkway
Suite 208
Merritt Island, Fl 32953
Find us on the web at: centralfloridafunctionalmedicine.com

Anju Usman, MD, FAAFP, ABIHM
True Health Medical Center
603 E Diehl Rd, Suite 135
Naperville, Illinois 60563
(630) 995-4242
www.truehealthmedical.com

Pure Compounding Pharmacy
Allergen free Preservative free prescriptions Chemical free prescriptions
603 E Diehl Rd Suite 131
Naperville, Illinois 60563
(630) 995-4300
www.purecompoundingpharmacy.com

James (Jack) Lyons-Weiler, PhD
CEO and Director, Institute for Pure and Applied Knowledge
Pittsburgh, PA
http://ipaknowledge.org

FOR MORE INFORMATION ON HOW TO PREVENT AUTISM:

Please visit my website: www.howtopreventautism.org
Or check my blog for recipes and wellness information www.daraberger.com
You can also see our health posts on my *How to Prevent Autism* Facebook page:
https://www.facebook.com/How-to-Prevent-Autism-738955156287184/
Visit me on twitter: PreventAutism@Dylanjakesmom